A PLUME BOOK

ABOUT WHAT WAS LOST

JESSICA BERGER GROSS graduated from Vassar College and received an MA in public affairs from the University of Wisconsin–Madison. She writes a column about international adoption for the *Literary Mama* online magazine, and teaches creative nonfiction at the Harvard Extension School. A longtime yoga student, her essays and articles have appeared in *Yoga International* and *Yoga Journal*, and on Salon.com and in other publications. She and her husband, Neil Gross, live in Cambridge, Massachusetts.

D1021190

About What Was Lost

20 Writers on Miscarriage,
Healing, and Hope

Edited by
Jessica Berger Gross

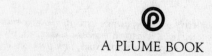

A PLUME BOOK

PLUME
Published by Penguin Group
Penguin Group (USA) Inc., 375 Hudson Street, New York, New York 10014,
U.S.A. • Penguin Group (Canada), 90 Eglinton Avenue East, Suite 700, Toronto,
Ontario, Canada M4P 2Y3 (a division of Pearson Penguin Canada Inc.) •
Penguin Books Ltd., 80 Strand, London WC2R 0RL, England • Penguin Ireland,
25 St. Stephen's Green, Dublin 2, Ireland (a division of Penguin Books Ltd.) •
Penguin Group (Australia), 250 Camberwell Road, Camberwell, Victoria 3124,
Australia (a division of Pearson Australia Group Pty. Ltd.) • Penguin Books India
Pvt. Ltd., 11 Community Centre, Panchsheel Park, New Delhi–110 017, India •
Penguin Books (NZ), cnr Airborne and Rosedale Roads, Albany, Auckland 1310,
New Zealand (a division of Pearson New Zealand Ltd.) • Penguin Books
(South Africa) (Pty.) Ltd., 24 Sturdee Avenue, Rosebank, Johannesburg 2196,
South Africa

Penguin Books Ltd., Registered Offices: 80 Strand, London WC2R 0RL, England

First published by Plume, a member of Penguin Group (USA) Inc.

First Printing, January 2007

10   9   8   7   6   5   4   3   2   1

Ⓟ REGISTERED TRADEMARK—MARCA REGISTRADA

LIBRARY OF CONGRESS CATALOGING-IN-PUBLICATION DATA

About what was lost : 20 writers on miscarriage, healing, and hope / edited by Jessica
Berger Gross.
    p. cm.
  Includes bibliographical references.
  ISBN-13: 978-0-452-28799-0
  1. Miscarriage—Psychological aspects. I. Gross, Jessica Berger.
  RG648.A26 2007
  155.9'37—dc22
                                                              20060240969

Printed in the United States of America
Set in Goudy

For Neil

Acknowledgments

This anthology wouldn't exist without my agent, Doug Stewart, at Sterling Lord Literistic, who believed in it (and me); Danielle Friedman at Plume, who edited the manuscript with care and grace; and my contributors, who so generously shared their stories and friendship. A special thank-you to my husband, Neil Gross, for his limitless love and support.

Contents

Introduction:
Behind the Bathroom Door

One Mother's Day, when I was a little girl living in Long Island, I went with my parents and two older brothers to visit my aunt Enid in her one-bedroom apartment in Queens. She was newly pregnant, not yet showing. Earlier that day, my uncle Peter, Enid's husband, had given her a Mother's Day card, which she shyly displayed on the coffee table. We snacked on peanuts and chocolate layer cake and watched a tennis match on television. All the adults in the room seemed relieved and I knew why. For as long as I could remember, I'd overheard my mother and her friends speaking in hushed tones about Enid's struggle to have a baby.

And then Enid disappeared into the bathroom and stayed for what seemed like much too long. Peter went to investigate. We heard Enid crying from down the hall. My parents quickly ushered us out, and without discussion we drove back home. I don't remember the word "miscarriage" having been spoken but it was obvious that something had gone wrong with the pregnancy, and that Enid's loss would be added to the long list of *things we don't talk about*. Poor Enid, I thought, and in the next moment I wished that whatever had happened to her in the bathroom would never happen to me.

Years later, at age thirty-one, it was me. I'd moved to Los Angeles with my husband, Neil, the year before, and we'd come across the name of an obstetrician in an article about prenatal yoga and natural childbirth. We'd done a little research and discovered he was one of the best in the city. I hadn't worried about the appointment, my first of the pregnancy, until the night before. I was young, healthy, and very morning-sick, which was supposed to be a good sign. For some reason, though, I couldn't sleep. Neil rolled over and reassured me that everything would be okay.

But the next morning, the news was bad. Staring up at an ultrasound screen in the doctor's office in Beverly Hills, I saw that there was no heartbeat, no fetus at all inside the embryonic sac. My pregnancy, at just eight and a half weeks, was over.

The next few weeks were a blur. I crawled into bed, turned on the television, and sobbed for days on end. I had dreamed about having a baby all my life, and in the last month had begun to fill in the details: the short list of literary French names I'd choose from, the infant massage classes we'd attend at my local yoga center, the chic Santa Monica baby store where we'd shop—and, eventually, the university town to which the three of us would move in search of a simpler life. At that time, unsure of myself in my new career as a writer, I had hung all my hopes on motherhood. The baby and I would spend our days together, making art, hanging out in the park, visiting my professor husband on campus during lunchtime, and developing the sort of intense bond I never had with my own mother.

The loss of the pregnancy shattered me. I missed my baby, all the more because we would never meet. I couldn't imagine ever dreaming such sweet dreams again. My pain was so deep, so bottomless, that at times I didn't want to go on.

I was too sad to talk to anyone, but Neil sent e-mails to our close friends about what had happened. Sympathy cards and e-mails and phone calls poured in. Most people didn't know what to say other than that they were sorry. A few told me about their own losses. My landlord's ex-wife had had two miscarriages before their son was born, and Neil's aunt had lost a pregnancy years ago, as well. Two of my childhood friends, recent mothers, had also lost first pregnancies. Neither had talked with me much about her grief at the time, but as I regained my ability to connect with the world, they began to open up.

It was a hard subject to discuss. Somewhere along the way we'd all picked up the idea that this wasn't something we should be so upset about. Our doctors had told us the same thing, that miscarriage was nature's way of ending a doomed pregnancy gracefully. The fact that we'd gotten pregnant in the first place meant that we could again. The best way to get over miscarriage, they advised, was to start trying to have another baby. But while both of my friends had gone on to have children, neither had finished grieving her miscarriage. Although Neil and I would start trying again a month later, my grief, too, remained, becoming a part of me. How long would the sadness last? Were we making too much of this?

In search of answers, I went back to the same stack of pregnancy books I had so eagerly consulted months before for relentlessly cheery advice on everything from a balanced prenatal diet to maternity underwear. But such books concentrate exclusively on healthy pregnancies; not wanting to scare readers, they offer little information on what might go wrong, or advice about how to handle the emotional fallout if it does.

In fact, the one piece of advice pertaining to miscarriage that these books do offer is that newly pregnant women should wait until the end of the tenuous first trimester to announce their pregnancy so that they will be spared the possible "embarrassment" and discomfort of sharing the sad news of a miscarriage. People, I've noticed, have taken this advice to heart, even developing superstitions around it. A close friend of mine, with my best interest at heart, was surprised when I revealed the news of my pregnancy in my fifth week. "Are you sure you should be telling me this now?" she asked. Don't tempt fate, the tone of her voice warned.

But here's the problem with keeping pregnancy a secret: If friends and relatives and coworkers and neighbors don't know about your pregnancy, how will they provide support if the worst *does* happen? And, besides, women who make it to their second trimester aren't protected from miscarriage occurring later on, or from the tragic loss of a baby during labor or soon afterward.

The more I thought about it, the more I realized that the notion of keeping one's pregnancy a secret for the first three months is just one aspect of a wider veil of secrecy surrounding miscarriage and pregnancy loss. I thought I was fairly knowledgeable about women's bodies—I'd taken my share of women's studies courses in college—but was shocked to discover that 20 to 25 percent of all pregnancies end in miscarriage. Why, then, doesn't anyone talk about it? Is it because we believe, somewhere deep down, that the inability to carry a baby to term reflects a moral failing on the part of the mother, as if she were somehow undeserving of motherhood? Was I less than fully feminine because I'd lost my baby? Was I in some way defective? These were the questions I kept asking myself in the days and weeks following my miscarriage, even though I knew such thoughts made no sense. In other moments, I wondered whether the lack of conversation about miscarriage might be a necessary by-product of the heated debate on abortion, with feminists like myself unwilling to publicly mourn the loss of a fetus for fear of giving legitimacy to pro-life views, and pro-lifers incapable of seeing miscarriage as anything other than God's plan? Or is it, more simply, part of a larger Western cultural pattern of avoiding any head-on confrontation with death and its emotional aftermath?

I've always found a particular kind of comfort in reading, so as I began to think more about these questions, it was only natural that I would search my favorite bookstores for anything about miscarriage. But I didn't find many books from which to choose. There were a couple of self-help volumes and a few more academic titles, but what I was craving were intimate stories about how other women had dealt with their losses and gone on to try (or not) again. Really, I wanted to know that I wasn't alone.

I'd hoped to return home with an armload of books, but instead I came away with an idea for a book of my own. In the collection that follows, twenty writers bravely and honestly share their stories of early love and loss, and reveal that with time and self-reflection, healing and hope are possible.

In collecting these essays I learned there are many ways a pregnancy can go wrong. Rachel Zucker, for example, was overwhelmed when she found out she was pregnant with twins, only to be told a few weeks later that one of the babies had disappeared in what is termed "vanishing twin syndrome." She writes about the uncomfortable mix of grief and relief she experienced. Many of the miscarriages described in the following pages are first-trimester ones, like mine. Andrea Buchanan woke up one morning late in her seventh week and realized she was bleeding. New to Philadelphia, without an OB, and with her husband stuck in a medical school class, she confirmed that she was having a miscarriage when, still bleeding, she took another pregnancy test and it came up negative. But not all pregnancy losses happen in the first three months. Sylvia Brownrigg's son Linnaeus was born prematurely at twenty-three weeks and died an hour later. She writes movingly about the delivery, about the short time she spent with her son, and about scattering his ashes near Lake Tahoe in the Sierras.

Sometimes women live with a pregnancy that has ended without their knowing it. When Miranda Field's morning sickness abated in her twelfth week, she also experienced it as a relief. "I don't know," she writes, that "the quiet child is dead. I'm happy no longer to be feeling sick." It's not until three weeks later that she found out the pregnancy was over. She needed to have a D and C—a dilation and curettage—immediately, or risk massive hemorrhaging. In the weeks that followed, she felt empty and alone.

The emotional complications of miscarriage are no less painful for an unplanned pregnancy. Jessica Jernigan, thirty and fresh from a breakup, discovered she was pregnant while living in a cabin in the mountains. Overjoyed, she decided she would be a single mom and was heartbroken when she miscarried at twelve weeks. Joyce Maynard, the mother of three grown children, lost an unplanned pregnancy much later in life. That she had already scheduled an abortion, at the urging of her then boyfriend, did nothing to take away her sadness.

The losses women experience through miscarriage, however, affect not only them, but their relationships with those they love. Rachel Hall struggled to explain to her five-year-old daughter, Maude, why her new sister or brother wouldn't be coming home after all. Julianna Baggott and her husband, David Scott, share an intimate conversation about their miscarriage and what it meant to them in light of the suicide of a close friend that occurred around the same time. Often, women who miscarry feel disconnected from their partners, however well-meaning they may be. Susanna Sonnenberg writes about twin losses, a terminated pregnancy followed by the miscarriage of a second pregnancy that was meant to make up for the abortion, and the emotional gap that opened between her and her husband when their efforts at consolation yielded heartbreak instead.

For some women, the mourning process may stretch out over many years, affecting choices, relationships, lives. Elizabeth Oness explores how she came to the conclusion, after two miscarriages, that her family of three was complete as it was. Her decision to stop trying to conceive made sense for her as mother and a writer, though it came with some sadness and regret. Likewise, Rochelle Jewel Shapiro, now a grandmother, still misses and mourns the baby she and her husband lost so many years ago.

Although such losses are never forgotten, I learned, while collecting these essays, that new love and life can help restore a sense of meaning and hope. Rebecca Johnson lost her son Luke, born fifteen weeks premature. After a second pregnancy ended in miscarriage, her son Simon was born and life began again. Caroline Leavitt went on to have a child after her miscarriage, too. She'll never stop thinking about the baby that was lost, but her son is nine now, "beautiful and smart and funny," and the day he was born was "the most profound experience of [her] life." Jen Marshall recounts her long and difficult struggles with infertility and how she miscarried after finally getting pregnant through in vitro fertilization. She eventually overcame the challenges of infertility, and is now the mother of twin boys, John and Reid.

Yet new babies are not the only thing that can make life feel worthwhile after a miscarriage. Pam Houston—who ultimately decided not to have children—rebounded from her miscarriage experience to embrace a life filled with work, friendship, love, dogs, and much travel and adventure. Over time, she has come to realize there are many ways she can express maternal love, whether it's traveling with her goddaughter or mentoring her writing students. New relationships may be formed around these losses, as well. Emily Bazelon and Dahlia Lithwick, legal journalists and editors, forged a friendship while exchanging a series of e-mails about their miscarriage experiences, a dialogue that touched many readers when it was published in *Slate*. And psychologist Susan O'Doherty used the years she spent dealing with multiple miscarriages to determine what she was meant to do with her life; now she is both a mother and a writer.

I found myself going through a similar process of self-discovery after my miscarriage. Forced to postpone motherhood, I threw myself into my work, my yoga practice, and learning how to be happy. As I wrap up work on this collection, I am excitedly awaiting news about the little girl my husband and I are adopting from India.

I've organized the pieces in this anthology into three sections. In the first, "Searching for Meaning," writers struggle to make sense of their miscarriage experiences and to understand them in the context of their personal biographies and the nature of women's lives today. In the second section, "In the Thick of It," contributors recount the difficult rush of the first few days, weeks, and months of a pregnancy loss—the doctors' waiting rooms, the ultrasounds, the D and Cs. Here, in the cracks and crevices of everyday experience, lie the realities of miscarriage, the traumas, and the tedious and terrifying moments that will never be forgotten. In the third section, "Mourning and Moving On," authors reflect on the long-term impact of miscarriage, on memory and acceptance.

I thank these women (and Julianna Baggott's husband, David Scott) for their openness, for being frank about their lives and the complex web of emotions surrounding birth and death. Speaking of things we are told to leave unsaid isn't easy. Not only have these writers opened a window into their most private lives, they write with eloquence and grace.

As I've collected these essays over the past two years, they have been my solace and many of the writers have become my friends. I hope this book provides a similar kind of comfort and companionship to women and their partners and loved ones in the aftermath of a pregnancy loss. And I hope, too, that it will serve as a starting point for more conversations, both private and public, about miscarriage, so that women and their partners won't have to go on grieving in silence.

Jessica Berger Gross
Cambridge, Massachusetts
May 2006

Editor's Note

Several of the following essays have been previously published; most appear here in slightly altered form. Andrea J. Buchanan's "Misconceptions" is taken from her book *Mother Shock: Loving Every (Other) Minute of It* (Seal Press) and expanded. A version of Dahlia Lithwick and Emily Bazelon's dialogue first appeared in *Slate* magazine. Pam Houston's "Pregnancy and Other Natural Disasters," now updated, was originally published in her collection *A Little More About Me* (W. W. Norton & Company). Rebecca Johnson's "Risky Business" was first published in *Vogue*.

PART I

~

Searching for Meaning

The First Baby

Caroline Leavitt

I like to think my pregnancy began in Notre Dame cathedral in Paris. I was there with my new husband on vacation, both of us in our southern forties, both writers, and the thing we both wanted most, beside each other, was a child.

I didn't know if I could get pregnant—something that worried me. I had been wild as a kid, and naïve. I believed a boyfriend who told me there was an herb that could safely abort any baby we might make, and agreed that as long as he came outside of me, I'd never get pregnant. Nothing had ever happened. Not with him, not with the boys I slept with whose condoms broke, not with my IUD that got infected and slipped out, not with the diaphragm. (I knew that old joke: What do you call people who use the diaphragm? *Parents.*) I hadn't given it much thought then, because a baby was the last thing on my mind.

But now was different. I wasn't a kid anymore. I was older. I had the right man and I yearned desperately for a baby. And because the noise from my biological clock was just about thundering, I knew I didn't have a lot of time. And so I stood there in the hazy golden light of Notre Dame and did what any good Jewish girl would do. I lit a candle and made a prayer: *Please. I want to have a baby. Please. Oh please.*

⁓

Two months later, I was pregnant.

You've never seen a mom-to-be like me. I glowed like the headlights on a highway. I beamed. Nothing bothered me. I know it was silly, but because of the Notre Dame candle, I felt protected somehow. I had read tons of pregnancy books, but I skipped the chapters about the things that could go wrong, because really, nothing would. Not with me. I was so lucky! I had no morning sickness! I could eat anything I wanted and have no cravings! My writing blossomed, fueled by my pregnancy, and I'd pat my belly and with a laugh I'd say, "This is my real work in progress. This is the most creative thing I've ever produced." Jeff would laugh, too. "I coproduced," he'd reply.

Even though I didn't show, I went out and spent a small fortune on pregnancy clothes, and every time I walked into my obstetrician's office I was smiling so hard he would burst out laughing. "You're the only one of my patients who never complains," he said. Every night Jeff and I lay in bed and imagined what it would be like with this new little heartbeat beside us.

But although we talked about it, we didn't tell anyone else. I was superstitious. I wanted to wait until the amniocentesis— four months away—when I would know what the sex of our child was, when we would be sure the baby was fine. In the meantime, I'd hide my belly in roomy shirts or flowing dresses. No one would know anything I didn't want them to know.

⌒

I was at the three-and-a-half-month point and was going for a checkup. Jeff was at a meeting, so I was going alone. It's funny, but I remember what I was wearing, an expensive black linen dress that hid the slight, tender swell that was my baby, and long dangling earrings. My hair rippling down my back. I loved my obstetrician, a warm funny guy named Steve who always joked and laughed with me, whom I had made promise he wouldn't dare go on vacation on my delivery day. I walked into the waiting room and smiled at Carol, his nurse. I sat down next to a woman with frizzy red hair and a huge belly. "Seven months," she said happily, patting her stomach. "Nearly four," I told her, stroking mine. And we bonded, just like that.

Today was a sonogram, the usual squirt of jelly on my belly, the vaginal wand at this stage, which would pick up the subtle *boom-boom-boom* of the baby's heartbeat. The baby's heartbeat! Was anything more wonderful? Usually, Steve, the nurse, and I all talked excitedly and swapped stories and jokes through the procedure, but this time, Steve suddenly stopped talking. Like dominoes, the nurse grew quiet, and then I got silent, too, until the whole room froze. "Digging for gold?" I blurted, and then I looked up and Steve glanced at his nurse who averted her eyes. "Steve?" I said. "Is everything okay?" And he looked at me and I felt a pulse of fear.

"I'm not getting a heartbeat," he said, and I sat up, suddenly dizzy. "I'm going to send you upstairs, to a better sono-gram," he told me. He patted my shoulder. "They should find the beat," he said. "You go up there and then come back down."

I dressed and walked upstairs, stunned and terrified, wish-ing for Jeff. Even if I called him now, he'd never be able to get there on time. As soon as I got to the top of the flight, wait-ing for me was a doctor I didn't know, frowning, impatiently saying my name. "There," he said, and pointed to a room, a long table, and another machine.

He squirted gel on my belly and turned on a computer. He ran a wand over my belly, muttering something to himself. There was a buzz from the machine, and then he tapped one finger on the screen to show me the long, flat green line, a deafening silence.

"What's that?" I asked.

"Dead," he said, and I bolted up.

"What?" I said, my voice cracking. "What did you say?"

"For a week already, it looks like. Maybe more."

I burst into tears, covering my face with my hands.

"Oh, for God's sake!" he scolded as if I had wet my pants in public. "Older babies than yours have died, you know!" And then he stormed out of the room and for the first time since I had gotten pregnant, I felt completely and devastatingly alone.

⌒

I cried getting dressed. I cried walking downstairs, and as soon as I saw Carol, I cried even harder, this time on her shoulder. I cried in Steve's office as he quietly talked to me.

"It's nature's way sometimes," he told me. "There's usually something terribly wrong with babies that die like that. Because of your age, it's probably Down syndrome."

"Wrong! Something wrong with my baby!" I cried.

"Look," he said gently, "we'll find out. We can do a test if you like. And it doesn't mean the next baby you might have won't be perfectly healthy."

The next baby! I nodded, my eyes pooling with tears. "I want the test," I said. "Please do the test."

He studied me for a moment. "The fetus won't expel," he said quietly. "We'll have to take it out. Think of it as a big D and C."

"When?" I asked.

"Tomorrow," he said. "First thing in the morning. Earliest time we can do it. We'll put you under and you won't feel a thing."

I walked out of the office into the waiting room, and this time, the redheaded woman I had joked with gave me one terrified look and then glanced away, refusing to meet my eyes.

❧

I hadn't brought my cell phone. Downstairs, I found a pay phone and called Jeff, weeping. And then, while I waited for him to come and get me, I made all the calls I had planned to make after the amniocentesis, only this time, they weren't celebratory announcements. There was no toast of fizzy apple juice instead of champagne, no laughter or whoops or jokes. I called my friend Linda who had a young son. I called my mother and my sister and left weeping messages and because

I was in a hospital, filled with crying people, surrounded by disaster, no one even looked twice at me. And then Jeff was suddenly there, and he was crying, too.

~

All that day, I lay in bed, unable to move. Jeff lay beside me, holding my hand, talking to me, but I felt as if I were under an anesthetic. I couldn't feel his touch. I couldn't really hear his voice. I used to keep my hand on my belly all the time, but now every time my fingers brushed the skin, they recoiled. My baby was dead, a punishment to me, and all I kept thinking was that I couldn't bear to be carrying it a second longer. I just wanted the operation over and done with so I didn't have to be reminded each time I took a breath.

I wasn't supposed to eat or drink anything but clear liquids before the operation. That morning, I sipped tea with dribbles of honey and clutched Jeff's hand and we went to the hospital for the surgery.

"Eat anything?" a doctor asked and I shook my head.

"Drink anything?"

"Tea with honey."

There was silence. The doctor sighed. "Tea with honey? You can't drink tea with honey!" He looked around and called over Steve, my doctor, who had just come in. He looked at me accusingly. "We can't do the operation today. She's had tea with honey."

Panicked, I stood up. I couldn't go another second with my dead baby inside of me—it was driving me mad, it was compounding my grief. "It was only a little honey!" I cried, though I knew it was spoonfuls. I didn't care—I didn't think that anything would happen, but the doctors all conferred, and then there was Steve and I grabbed his hand. "I can't wait another day," I said, my voice raw. "Please. Please." And then he studied me carefully, and he must have seen how desperate I was, how on the edge, because he said okay.

I remember waking from the operation, and feeling suddenly so alone. There was no body to hold. No name. And although that baby was the size of a pea, like the proverbial princess, I felt the loss. It wasn't there anymore. There was just me. I had lost my baby the moment the doctor told me there was no heartbeat, but now that the baby was no longer inside of me, it felt like a new, second loss. "We'll do some tests, find out what happened," Steve told me. "You go home and rest. Then come see me in a week and we'll talk."

I went back to bed, though I couldn't sleep. I couldn't read or watch TV or eat. I lay beside Jeff, holding hands and crying and feeling dead inside. The doctor called to tell me the fetus had had severe Down syndrome, that it was so damaged it couldn't have lived. "It's a blessing," he told me, but all I could think of was why didn't it feel like one? Friends called, telling me stories, comforting me, making me feel a little less alone. My friend Anna started crying, too, because she had had a miscarriage two years before. Lindy, an acquaintance who intimidated me, whom I barely knew, called and said, "Oh, tulip, I'm so sorry," with such warmth in her voice, that we became immediate and fast friends. My mother and sister called twice a day with stories and bad jokes, and sometimes they just listened to me telling the story of my miscarriage, over and over, as if by telling it I might rewrite the script, I might change what had happened.

⟶

But if friendships were one thing, work, and going back to it, was another.

I was—and am—a novelist and a journalist, but I couldn't concentrate enough on writing to even think of turning on my computer. The work in progress I had cared most about, my baby, was gone, and I had no heart left to try and create anything else. I'd put my writing aside, give myself six months, if I had to. But unfortunately, it wasn't just my creative work I had to tend to. Like most writers, Jeff and I also had steady jobs in addition to our writing, fairly mindless jobs that could supply the extra financial benefits (and health insurance) we needed. But while Jeff's job was pleasant, mine was in an angry corporate beehive, a video catalog company where I wrote about movies, a job that originally had been lots of fun. The man who had hired me, thrilled to have "a real writer" on board, had left, and the climate had since soured, to the point that I was now viewed with suspicion. Just months earlier, when my novel got a rave in the *New York Times*, I had pinned the review to my bulletin board; two hours later, I was hauled into my new boss Tom's office. I had figured he was going to congratulate me, that he'd share in my amazed joy, but instead he jabbed his finger at the review. "Any mistakes here, people are going to pin them on you," he had warned. "They'll think you're thinking about your novel and not videos. Take the review down. And don't talk about it. Be more of a company person."

I tucked the review in my desk and kept opening the drawer to gaze at it. But after that, while I'd talk about my writing life with coworkers who asked, I never again volunteered information, and I never talked about being a novelist—or anything personal—with Tom again.

Until now, when I had to call him and tell him I needed a week off.

⁓

I thought of my office environment, the way some people talked and whispered and laughed about everyone else's business. I thought of the few coworkers whom I liked, and how, if I told them, they'd be so sympathetic, I would burst into tears and never stop. I didn't talk about my writing life at work, and I wouldn't talk about this, either. Better, I thought, for no one at work to know anything about what had happened. Better for me to come back and sit at my desk, anesthetized by the pages and pages of copy I'd churn out. I'd lie to Tom. I'd tell him I had the flu.

Tom answered on the first ring. And then, to my horror, before I could even start to get my lie out, I started to cry. I was so raw, the words tumbled out. "I had a miscarriage," I blurted. And to my surprise, Tom became grave and sympathetic. "You take however long you need," he said.

"I need to come back as soon as I can," I told Tom. "I need to lose myself in work, but I don't want anyone to know. It's too personal—too painful."

"God, don't worry!" he assured me, his voice richly sympathetic. "I'll see to it that everyone thinks you have bronchitis."

He promised me he wouldn't say a word.

Two hours later, Nancy, an art director from work, called, her voice rushed. "I'm so sorry about your miscarriage," she said, and my breath stopped.

"How did you know?" I asked slowly, trying not to sound upset. "Who told you?"

"Tom," she said, and then she hesitated. "Listen, I think you should know, he's telling everyone. And he's making jokes about it. Older-mother stuff. Everyone knows. Everyone."

Stunned, I hung up. I had trusted Tom, had given him the benefit of a doubt, and he had betrayed me in the cruelest way possible. I could accuse him myself, but could I trust that he wouldn't make fun of that act as well? I immediately called Diane, the head of Human Resources, a burly woman who had never done more than nod at me in the hall. Talking to her meant more people at work would know, but I had to stop Tom.

"We'll hold a big meeting with all of us, including Tom's boss, to discuss it," Diane said.

I wrapped the phone cord tightly about my wrist. "I don't want to talk about any of this anymore!" I insisted. "I just want it to end. Can't *you* just talk with him?"

There was an odd silence. "These are serious charges," she said. "Are you thinking of suing for invasion of privacy? Do you have a lawyer?"

No, I told her. No, no, no.

⁓

A week later, I went back to work. I had no idea what I was going to do, though different scenarios kept running through my mind. I'd confront Tom and he'd apologize profusely. I'd confront Tom and he'd fire me on the spot. I'd say nothing and if people looked at me as if I were an exhibit to be stared at, I'd simply ignore them. Everything would be fine. Everything would be disaster. "Call me every hour," Jeff had told me. "And come home if you have to. Quit. We'll find some other health insurance. We'll figure something out."

As soon as I walked into the office, I felt my bones turning to water. Two people passed me in the hall, quickly averting their eyes, and I had to stop and lean against the wall, shutting my eyes, breathing deeply so I wouldn't weep. There were three messages on my machine from Diane in Human Resources. "We need to have that big meeting," she said curtly. There were twelve messages from friends. "I know this is going to be hard," one of them said. People stumbled awkwardly into my office and patted my shoulder. "At least you didn't know the baby," Christine, an art director, said. "I mean, at least it wasn't a real baby yet. Three months is nothing." Sam, in Marketing, said, "You'll get over it, it happened early." And Julie in Sales, who I had previously liked, said, "God, that's what happens when you try to have a baby past forty." I nodded numbly, because what good would it do to snap back at her? I got up and saw Tom walking toward me and I turned abruptly away from him because I knew that whatever he had to say I didn't want to hear. I went into the ladies' room and sat in a stall, staring blankly at the door, unable to move.

The world was full of babies. I couldn't get on the subway without seeing a mother smiling dreamily at her child. At restaurants kids rapped their spoons, babbled, and waved their hands at me, so sweetly I had to look away. And sometimes, God help me, I would stare at pregnant women and think: *It could happen to you.*

But help came. Jo, who had been one of my best friends since college, phoned from Santa Fe and just listened quietly while I cried. Another friend, Jane, told me how hard her own miscarriage had been, and how after she had miscarried her doctor had told her she could never get pregnant again because he now saw she had a blockage in her fallopian tubes, that she'd need an operation to clear it. The day of the operation, she had bronchitis and had to cancel it, which turned out to be a lucky break because she was pregnant with her daughter. "You got pregnant once," she told me. "You can get pregnant again."

My friend Peter showed up at my house. We'd been buddies for more than ten years, had nursed each other through bad dates, deaths, illness, and firings, and no one, except for Jeff, could make me laugh as much as he could. As soon as I saw him, I flung my arms around him and cried. "I brought you something," Peter told me and handed me a package. "Look, all of my friends think I'm nuts to do this. They think I'm cruel. They say, how can you give her this? But I keep telling them, oh no, she'll love this." He hesitated. "Hope I'm right."

I opened it up. It was a small handmade book. It had a heavy red paper cover, white creamy pages. "Look at the title," Peter urged. *Smart Answers for Dumb Questions*, it said. I opened the book. On the left-hand side of every page, Peter had written out one of the terrible remarks made to me. On the right-hand side was a funny, nasty response. For "At least you didn't know the baby," the response was, "Yeah, and if I had, I know he would have hated you!" For "At least it wasn't a real baby yet," Peter had scribbled, "Yeah, and you're so insensitive you aren't a real person!" I started to laugh at page three, the first time since the miscarriage, and by page six I was laughing so hard the tight coil in my belly loosened. I read that book every day for a month.

If I couldn't forget completely, people at work could. Gradually, they turned to other gossip and I settled back into a routine.

⁓

I got pregnant again almost immediately. This time, there was no magical candle, but there was pure, exact science, courtesy of an expensive ovulation kit. Jeff and I were both worn out and dozing through the sex, but I knew the time was perfect, and I kept waking him up and urging him into sex again, into completion, though I was rough and sore and dry and emotionally wounded, and he was exhausted. I stayed up with my legs crunched up against my chest, holding that baby in, willing that life to stick.

And it did.

⁓

This pregnancy was different. This time Jeff came to every doctor's appointment. This time we weren't going to tell

anyone anything, not even after the amnio, not until I
showed so much it would be too obvious to lie. I wore my big
shirts and roomy dresses and if anyone suspected enough to
ask if I was pregnant, I shook my head. "Just eating too
much," I'd say with a smile. When I reached the three-and-
a-half-month mark, the time when I had lost the first baby, I
grew quiet. Every time I peed, I searched my panties for a spot
of blood. I put my hands protectively over my belly. I prayed:
please, please, please. But this baby seemed to take. To hold on
fast, almost as if he knew what was at stake for me.

"Doing great," Steve told me at every visit. I held my
breath through the amnio. Jeff and I watched the blurry image of the baby swimming across the screen, and when Steve
asked if we wanted to know the sex, we nodded. "Boy," he
said. Boy! The baby had a sex! "We have to name him," I told
Jeff, because I knew that naming him would give my son
more presence; it anchored him more to life. "Max," I said. "I
want to call him Max."

Five and a half months into the pregnancy, I finally
popped, transforming, grown big with baby, and exuberant, I
told my family, my friends, the people at work. "This time's
for keeps!" everyone said, and though that was the one thing
I so desperately wanted, I couldn't help not being sure.

Filled with joy and hope, I still never totally relaxed, because
every new thing that happened with this pregnancy reminded
me of the first one. This time I read—no, I memorized—all the
chapters about all the things that could go wrong. I was fluent
in disaster words like eclampsia and PROM (premature rup-
ture of membranes), and I wore talismans and necklaces, and

every day I sang the Beatles' "I Will" to my baby. I took ridicu-
lously good care of myself, and the day he was born was the
most profound experience of my life.

~

After Max was born, people said things to me like, "See?
Maybe you had to lose that first baby so this special boy could
make his appearance." Coworkers said, "Now you can forget
the past!" No one wanted to talk about the first baby, no one
wanted to give it any sort of marker. And then, one evening,
my friend Jo called to congratulate me about Max. Her voice
grew low as she said, "I know you'll always consider the other
baby your first." And I cried not just because I knew she was
right, but because I finally felt that someone had heard me,
that someone understood.

Max is nine years old now. Beautiful and smart and funny.
And yes, sometimes when Jeff and I are in the midst of talking about what a great child we have, and how thrilling it is
to watch him grow, we talk, too, about that first baby. What
would it have been? A little girl? A little boy? What would
that child have been like? I keep thinking of it, the poor little thing, severely damaged by Down syndrome, and how I
could have loved it anyway. "You would have had to abort,"
people told me, and the one thing I most thank God for is
that I never had to make that decision because, as pro-choice
as I am, I don't know if I could have had an abortion. Once
you start loving something, once you invest it with personality and presence, how can you ever let it go?

But the yearning, the grief, never totally goes away. It's

there under the daily happinesses, the joy of a husband and another child. I mark off that baby's birthday every year. I grieve for that little soul. And sometimes I apologize to it, not because I believe I'm responsible, but because it never got to live. It never got the chance to be a real person. We never got to really know each other. It wasn't just the death of a baby, it was the death of hope, "The thing with feathers," as Emily Dickinson said, and it—and I—never had a chance to soar.

Misconceptions

Andrea J. Buchanan

" 'A happy man leads a long life.' What is that? That's a statement, not a fortune," said Ben.

We were out after work, having Chinese on the Upper West Side, me, my friends Liz and Ben, and my husband, Gil. "Wait, look at mine," said Liz. " 'Live life well and be happy.' What is *that?*"

"That's more of a directive, don't you think?" I said. I cracked open my cookie and unfolded the fortune. As I read it, I felt a rush of warmth flood my face.

"What's yours?" asked Ben.

" 'Your secret desire to completely change your life will manifest.' "

"Impressive!"

Gil held out his tiny piece of fortune-cookie paper with a bemused smile. He looked a little smug, so I knew he had something good. He cleared his throat and read his fortune aloud: " 'You are the greatest person in the world.' "

"Oh my god! You win!" said Liz.

"Hand it over," said Ben, angling for a look. I glanced at it as Gil reached across the table. He wasn't making it up; the fortune really said that.

Ben laughed when he read it. "Oh yeah, you win."

I smiled and laughed along with everyone else, but I knew that I was the real winner of the best fortune cookie contest.

Your secret desire to completely change your life will manifest.

I was going to have a baby.

⁓

I wasn't actually pregnant then, but I had been contemplating the idea with an intensity that surprised me. Gil and I had been married nearly three years. I was twenty-six, he was thirty. We were at that point where not only the in-laws inquired about the possibility of children. Friends of ours had announced recently over dinner that they were going to be parents; couples we knew from college sent us baby shower invitations; people we met at parties asked us if we were thinking about having kids. The idea of having a family had begun to seem less like a scene from someone else's grown-up life than I had previously imagined.

True, Gil was the one who would spy a cute baby sitting with its mother on the subway and nudge me, smiling. I smiled at the concept of cute babies, too, but for me, imagining what life would be like with a baby was too overwhelming to be realistic about, so I approached the notion as indirectly as possible. Sitting in my office at work, I'd envision a bassinet in the corner, a cooing baby kicking at an overhead mobile while I edited galleys and talked on the phone. That seemed doable, right?

A few months after that night in the Chinese restaurant, we moved to Philadelphia. Gil was beginning medical school at Penn after a career on Wall Street, and I was able to convince the magazine I worked for to let me telecommute and work from home in Philly. With Gil having the life of a student, and my work being home-based, we thought the time might be right to manifest that secret desire to completely change our lives. We began, as couples obliquely say when the topic of children is broached by strangers, "trying."

Soon after our move, and soon after the "trying" began, I found myself unusually stressed and fragile. I was weepy over commercials, shaky and dizzy if I skipped breakfast, prone to sobbing over a paper jam in my printer or a fax that failed to go through. I cried on the phone to the production manager over a typo I had missed. Finally, realizing that in addition to all that hypersensitivity I had also missed my period, I took a home pregnancy test: two lines. Positive.

In a matter of days after taking the test, my body already seemed to be changing. Besides feeling an emotional sensitivity, I was queasy, yet hungry—no, ravenous—all the time; my breasts were incredibly sore; I was already gaining weight, changing in shape.

After a week or two, flush with excitement, and against the conventional wisdom to wait a few months to announce the good news, we told Gil's parents. The next day, I lost the baby.

I have always been terrible at keeping secrets.

I woke up early that morning and discovered I was bleeding. As the morning progressed, the bleeding grew worse, and I knew, though I didn't want to know, that it was over. A few hours later, shaky and crying, I used the extra home pregnancy test from the pack I'd gotten seven weeks before. I let it sit for two minutes, which felt like two hours, as I bled, the test's window an empty reproach.

Still new to town, I hadn't even set up an appointment to see an OB-GYN. New also to the endeavor of pregnancy, I had no idea whether I needed to go to the hospital or simply let things happen as they happened. My husband was unreachable, sitting in some med-school classroom somewhere, diligently scribbling notes as he listened to his professor lecture on embryology.

I remembered that one of Gil's good friends from college, who, unlike him, had taken the direct route to becoming a doctor, was working as a physician in town, so I tracked her down. I called the hospital where I thought she worked, somehow managed to talk a nurse into giving me her emergency pager number, managed to wait until she finally called me back, and then choked out the words to communicate to her what was happening.

I asked her what I should do, and she told me what I already knew: I was losing the pregnancy. She told me to rest, to call her back if the bleeding got worse. I wept over the phone, sobbing that I couldn't understand what was happening, or *why* it was happening. I told her that even though it had been only a few hours since the bleeding began, I was already starting to lose my "pregnancy feeling"—no more swollen breasts, no more nausea, no more.

"I know," she told me. And as it sunk in that she meant more than just sympathy, that she really *knew*, she repeated it. "I know."

How could she know? Then she told me her story: It had happened to her, too. She had never told anyone else, aside from her partner, because she was not married, and to say that her very traditional family would have been unsupportive was an understatement. Her miscarriage at eight weeks was a grief she experienced in private, and she understood even more than I did at that moment the difficulty of keeping that grief private for others' sake, the sadness of living as though you are not secretly in mourning. She told me how difficult it was for her to reconcile her understanding as a medical professional of miscarriage as a common occurrence with her profoundly raw, emotional reaction to losing the pregnancy—even though she had contemplated terminating it. My husband's friend and I shared our stories with each other, and by the time we hung up, I felt a little less alone.

⁓

As strange as it had been to be pregnant—feeling my body taken over by uncontrollable hunger and emotion—it was stranger to no longer be pregnant. The bleeding continued like a long, heavy period. Every once in a while I would feel nauseated and it would hit me that it wasn't because I was growing a life inside me but because I was losing one. When I would get an occasional hunger pang, it would remind me of the intensity of my hunger during the previous few weeks.

My boss happened to call me that afternoon, while I was struggling to process everything I was feeling. I couldn't pull myself together enough to sound professional on the phone, and I told her, through tears, what had happened. I was jarred out of my grief by her oddly upbeat response: "That's great— at least you know you can get pregnant."

What is she talking about? I thought. But then she explained: She had been trying to conceive for years with no luck. From her perspective, even a spontaneously aborted pregnancy was a positive sign. "This one wasn't meant to be; it was off; there was something wrong with it," my boss told me. "Just be glad your body knew what to do with it. Don't be sad about it, just try again. Really, it's for the best."

Talking to my husband's friend and my boss, I was struck by the personal revelations suddenly shared as a result of my own loss, the stories these women seemed to have that I never knew before, the dawning realization that getting pregnant and having a baby was not as straightforward as I'd imagined.

What if it happened again? What if I got pregnant for a second time, only to miscarry at eight weeks, just like this time, just like Gil's friend? What if, like my boss, I found that I was unable to get pregnant? What if I was never meant to be a mother at all?

When my husband came home from his classes that day and found me still on the couch, my face blotchy and tear stained, I told him what happened and said, "I don't know how people do this. I don't know if I can do this again."

He held me and let me cry.

~

A week after my miscarriage, Liz came from New York to visit. We spent a lot of time just walking around town, exploring the neighborhoods, talking about people we both used to work with and the restaurants we used to go to, including the Chinese place where I'd gotten that fortune.

I talked about the miscarriage—I needed to explain it to her, to myself, to process it. And yet it was awkward. The new physical separation from each other—me in Philadelphia, her in New York—seemed a metaphor for the distance between our experiences. I felt as though in getting pregnant, I had gone somewhere she hadn't, and that even though I'd lost the pregnancy and returned to being, like her, a non-pregnant woman, the distance was still there. I felt apologetic, as though I'd tried something extravagant (look at me, I'm married, I'm having a baby!) and failed. There were things I couldn't explain to her, things she didn't know, and there was no way I could go back to a time when I didn't know them, either. She listened to me say what I needed to say, and she reassured me the way a good friend does, offering sympathy and a completely unfounded assurance that next time everything would work out fine.

I didn't know how to tell her about my grief, about how helpless I felt, how powerless, how the whole experience called into question a realm of my physical body I'd taken for granted and never considered before.

Our long walk through town took us to the Philadelphia Museum of Art, where we admired the Van Goghs and the Eakinses, and I lost myself for a little while in the satisfaction of looking at beautiful things. Before we left, we hit the contemporary wing, where there was an installation on display.

"Oh my god, look at that," Liz said, pointing. I was caught off guard by what I saw.

It was a room full of what looked like fruit, oranges and bananas and grapefruit carefully laid out on the floor. Museum patrons were allowed to interact with the exhibit, and the sight of casually dressed tourists tiptoeing around the fruit, careful not to disturb it, peering closely and in some cases taking pictures, made me laugh out loud.

Then, as we came closer, I saw that it wasn't just fruit strewn about the room, it was *dead* fruit. Rotten bananas, and oranges and grapefruits gone soft. As I walked even closer, I saw that the fruit was not merely decayed: Each piece had been carefully hollowed out, the rotted inner flesh scooped and scraped away, and the outside peels stitched up to make the fruit appear whole again. Some were sewn up with thick, brightly colored yarn, the kind used to tie bows in little girls' braids. Some were held together with thread in fanciful cross-stitch patterns. Some were laced with surgical stitches. Some had glittery buttons, some had jaunty bows. As I finally entered the room, I found myself crouching to the ground with the rest of the tourists, unable to stop myself from touching the yarn and bows and buttons, the futile attempts to infuse the dead things with life again.

Liz put her hand on my shoulder as I sat on the floor of the exhibit, unable to stop myself from crying. The installation, she told me, was called *Strange Fruit*.

In those days I thought a lot about in-between places. The spaces between the dead fruit where people walked in the exhibit; the pregnancy I had lost on its way between being a clump of cells and a beating heart; the in-between place I floated in, being not a mother, but no longer someone who had never been pregnant. I couldn't go back to my life before, somehow erasing the memory of what those intense few weeks were like in my body. But I wondered, could I go on? Could I try to get pregnant again knowing what I knew, that it could be lost, quite literally, in a heartbeat?

I pored the Internet looking for more stories like the ones I'd heard from the friends I'd spoken to about my miscarriage. I read the bulletin boards for women dealing with pregnancy loss, both to gorge myself on details and satiate my desire for proof of other people's experience with what I'd gone through. I read about people who'd lost their pregnancies earlier than I had and grieved harder; I read tragic stories about people who'd lost babies even after a full nine months' gestation. I read these stories obsessively, as if to inoculate myself, as if reading the most heartbreaking tale could prevent something similar from happening to me the next time I attempted motherhood, if I dared.

I posted on the bulletin boards and introduced myself. I told my tale. I joined the club. Soon I knew the stories of everyone there; I knew what the positive and negative signs were in early pregnancy; I knew what tests were recommended;

I knew when it was safe to try again after miscarrying once, twice, even three times. I felt armed with knowledge and comforted by the fact that if I did try again and fail, I had someplace to go, somewhere I could mourn and have my desperate grief understood.

⁓

Two weeks after my miscarriage Gil and I went to a friend's vocal recital in New York. I made small talk with everyone, never letting on about what had happened inside my body. I scanned the crowd for women, mothers, grandmothers, wondering how many might have had a story like mine. How many of us had invisibly nurtured our own strange fruit? How many of us had stitched up our grief with optimism? How many of us had had a secret desire to completely change our lives? And how many of us had been surprised by the kind of change that came our way?

On the way home, I helped Gil study for his molecular biology class by reading him his lecture notes, a strange, polysyllabic vocabulary of reticula and hemopoiesis and mesenchymal something-or-others. I read aloud for the entire two-hour drive, and at some point in the middle of the B-cells chapter I felt a distinct pain on the lower right side of my body, near my hip and about where my right ovary would be, according to the pictures I'd seen in his medical books.

I'd never had pain around the time of ovulation before, but I'd read about mittelschmerz and I had a fair idea that this dull aching, this tightness, was the sensation of an egg's being released, a message from my body that it was time again. The sensation lasted almost the whole evening, through the rest of the car ride, through our having sex, through dinner with a friend, through the walk home. I felt like the pain was deliberate, a message, someone tapping me on the shoulder and whispering, *It's time for me to be born.*

Two weeks later, I was pregnant again. This time I did not let myself map out my pregnancy the way I had the first time, writing into my calendar what my due date would be, or imagining how I would look in maternity clothes, or planning what I would say to my boss when it was time to apply for leave. I kept my hopes small, and limited my excitement to cautious postings on the Internet bulletin boards, where I graduated from the "Dealing with Loss" board to the one titled "Pregnant After Loss."

I traded e-mails with a woman who had miscarried a week before me and had gotten pregnant again a week before me. We kept each other focused on staying positive, exchanging updates on our developing symptoms, scanning our bodies for signs that our new pregnancies would work out. I called an OB-GYN my husband's doctor friend had recommended and was given an appointment a few weeks away. The delay seemed like a lifetime. The community of women online kept me company during my wait.

At my first ultrasound, at seven weeks, roughly around the same time I had miscarried the first pregnancy, I was half convinced they were playing a videotape of someone else's visit, so foreign did it seem that there could really be a living thing inside me. I was worried that all we would find was an empty sac, and at first that was all I could make out on the small screen, without my glasses. But as the picture began to take shape, I could see a little piece of fuzz clinging to the top of the gestational sac. The doctor said, "There's your baby!" and zoomed in closer. All of a sudden that little fuzz was pulsing with life; we could see the whole shape of it flashing with its heartbeat. My husband squeezed my hand hard and I started to tear up from the realization that it was real, from the relief of finding it to be real, from the sheer terror of it being real.

Then the doctor asked us if we wanted to hear the heartbeat. At first, there was only silence as the tech tuned the equipment, and I was sure I wouldn't be able to hear anything over the sound of my own heart, but after a few minutes the whole room was enveloped in sound: *whoosh-whoosh, whoosh-whoosh*. The doctor took some measurements and then looked around inside, checking my ovaries. He found the corpus luteum on the right, which meant that the egg came from the right ovary, exactly where I'd felt that surprising pain. We left the appointment with our shiny little ultrasound picture, the first picture of our first baby, proof that it had really happened, that it was really there.

I kept that picture with me like a talisman, looking at it every time I was dogged by the fear that this pregnancy, too, would be lost. I felt the tenuous nature of my endeavor, the unsettling knowledge that at any moment it could be taken from me.

When we go out for Chinese food now, my dining partners are not much interested in the tradition Gil and I have of critiquing our fortune-cookie fortunes. In fact, one of them is offended by the very notion of a cookie that is not in any way composed of two round chocolate halves sandwiching a white, fluffy center, and the other would gladly eat the fortune itself if not for my watchful eye. My children pick up rice with their fingers, ask for beverages they won't drink, charm the waitstaff into giving them strange-tasting Chinese candy. Our meals are bolted down rather than savored over adult conversation, the better to finish our food before a critical meltdown point is reached. We are a chaotic, fast-moving, loud bunch, drawing smiles from some patrons and perturbed frowns from others, depending on the emotional integrity of the kids that day, which itself seems to depend on the alignment of the planets, the stars being in the right place, the alchemy of a decent interval between previous meals and the natural luck of a good day.

This is what I know now that I didn't when I first looked to my fortune to tell me what life with children would bring: how much of it is luck, from the ability to become pregnant in the first place to the kind of temperament your child will have once she is born. Now that I am a parent, I am still looking for signs along the way, messages which I can take to mean I am on the right path, doing the best that I can. But I am no longer certain that the future they augur is a definite one, or even the one I think they mean.

My misconception, my miscarriage the first time around, was an abrupt introduction to the pure essence of parenting: the sheer chance of it all. The intensity, the joy, the grief, the fear of loss. The incontrovertible fact that the secret life you have created is simply out of your hands, beyond your control, beyond the scope of any other experience. It readied me, in ways I could not know until I was finally there, for motherhood, for the powerful rush of love and other overwhelming emotions, the depth and breadth of which I mistakenly thought I already knew.

Twins

Susanna Sonnenberg

Seven women started training at the abortion clinic that Monday, our chairs pulled in close to the conference table, our attention better tuned than it had ever been in college. The executive director thanked us for our underpaid commitment and gave a brief history of the clinic, its newly built facility having just opened after an arsonist razed the building two years before. She spoke frankly about the threats associated with the job. "I want to know why you're here," she said. "You have to really want to do this." We went around the table, each of us giving her reason. One woman had worked at a rape crisis hotline for years, aware that she had a gift for helping others face difficulties. Someone else was doing her practicum for the local university's psych program. I was here, I said, because I knew what a bad abortion felt like and wanted to be part of something better.

For four days we reviewed the biology of reproduction and conception, ovulation, and embryonic stages. We debated pregnancy options, rehearsing ways to explore them with our clients. We unpacked every meaning in "pro-choice" and

"mother" and read through the state's abortion-related legis-
lation. We picked apart the informed-consent form and drilled
evacuation routes and escort security. We spent one day on
birth control methods, the long table heaped in the center
with diaphragms, cervical caps, pill packets, and condoms,
with vaginal dams, sponges, and intra-uterine coils. The doctor came in and explained the procedure, naming the instruments he used. We toured the exam rooms, switched on the
vacuum aspirators, learned how to open the sterile packs
without breaking sterility. Saturated with knowledge, we
learned that the body intends so ferociously to become pregnant that we are almost powerless to stop it; only by slim luck
and great effort do we ensure another month with a period.
On Friday, the lab technician had us pee in cups and test our
urine on the pregnancy dipsticks. It was an exercise in tech-
nique, but I let my results be known and showed off the only
stick that had the double bars of pink darkened across its
window. I was pregnant. The other women clapped and gathered close.

This was not my first pregnancy with my husband. Three
months into our marriage, I told Christopher I needed a pregnancy test and walked into the downtown Planned Parenthood, which provided them for free. We were stunned. It's
not like we were college freshmen or oblivious drunken kids.
Since our first lovemaking two years before we always knew
what we were doing. We had intimate knowledge of a half
dozen birth control methods. We'd been using a cervical cap
which, we knew, didn't fit every woman, was tricky to place
properly, and was subject to being knocked off the cervix by

certain positions, but only other people made dumb mistakes. Careful and responsible, *we* had not wanted to get pregnant, not even a little bit. How would a pregnancy fit into our precious isolation, our primal love, new marriage? For two years the world had been made by us, spun around our bed by passion and intimacy, a world as complete as our dinner table with its two settings. We did not have room for someone else.

The accidental pregnancy cracked us open. Pregnancy, I had imagined, would make two people closer, but this physical rumor sliced through our center with quick, deft accuracy. For two days we sat with the news, waiting as if for someone else to make our decision and hand it to us. We talked and talked, made halfhearted jokes, cried. One day we pretended we would have the baby, and I felt splendid with nature and dazzled by the identity of me as a mother. The next day we pretended that we'd agreed to an abortion, and Christopher relaxed.

We arrived at the silent understanding that his unreadiness to be a father trumped my thrill. To survive as a couple— newly married and still fragile—we needed to end this pregnancy. This was my first insight that the marriage itself had an identity, distinct from either of ours. The big, bossy marriage mocked our idea that together we knew what we were doing.

"We choose abortion," I told the counselor at Planned Parenthood, a new "we" in my vocabulary. She noted my reasons—relationship, money, time—and pointed me to the signature line of the consent form. We. But I couldn't unknow what was going on in my bones and blood. A few days later I underwent the D and C. My body's brilliant trick undone, a loneliness carved itself into my marriage.

Christopher, meanwhile, came to see the possibilities, could now feel the shifting of roles into parenthood. My body had rendered the abstract concrete for him, and he thanked me. But I felt betrayed—by that clinic, by him, by nature—and my anger permeated the walls of our house, the sheets of our bed. It was an empty anger, tinged with hard jokes aimed to hurt him. I watched him figure out that he was ready to want children as I struggled with the awareness that maybe I didn't.

During the next months we talked, and didn't talk, about having a baby, rolling the subject back and forth, feeling out the contradictions. One day in summer Christopher pulled off the road into a dusty alcove of a canyon, the ground orange and soft with silty earth. He'd been quiet throughout the drive, and we got out of the car. He had his arm around my shoulder. He was smiling.

"Would you have that baby now?" he asked.

"Yes," I said, flooded with a delight of unfamiliar purity. We found a bookstore in the next town and bought What to Expect When You're Expecting, feeling renewed in love and confident with our decision as we paid. Later, though, again quiet in the car, I thought, "Not that baby. That baby's gone for good." It was the having and the not having, the tug of wanting and not wanting that would define pregnancy for me after that.

We put off making love. The sex would be different, and we were shy with intention, didn't know how we wanted it. I walked around with a knot in my chest that flared nervous and excited and sick, the emotions of a locked-in commitment.

Then we made love. At the moment that had always been reserved for birth control—one of us off to the bathroom with its cold floor or giving a quick tear at the foil packet—we realized that nothing compelled us to pause. We didn't need to suspend excitement, and we dared our bodies to take over. I felt a delicious giving up that had never been anticipated by the common surrenders of sex before. A warmth of love and purpose spread over my skin, my being. We waited. Every day I made love to my husband with purpose and concentration, with silent incantations and magical thinking: if I take off all my rings and my necklace, if I shower first, if I don't wear perfume, if we light four candles, if we make love at night, if we make love in the morning, then, then, then.

A few weeks later I used a drugstore test, spending the money to buy myself privacy this time. I reread the tiny words on the box until I knew the directions cold. Then I watched the positive result emerge, my eyes tricking me a dozen times in the space of a minute. I am, I'm not, I am. *I am.* Pressing my breasts for soreness, I looked in the bathroom mirror, and I saw myself as an outline, a container. Christopher wasn't home yet, and the news—divine, big, magnificent—was mine. I was the only one who knew, and I didn't want to share it with the person who took so long to decide. But that reaction was only a flicker, a stinginess I pushed away. He came home, I told him, and he was truly happy. We were more than pregnant: We were truly having a baby.

So much happened then. I called every friend, people I'd been out of touch with for months, and never tired of the exclamation, "I'm going to have a baby!" Christopher started graduate school to become a therapist (real family, real profession), and I started counseling at the clinic. Our life felt proper, our steps essential.

Now I had clients. When I closed the door to the counseling room, I left my concerns in the hall, left my pregnancy outside, the room big enough for just one of us to plumb her body. The stories of choice were never the same and never adhered to a comfortable narrative. But, like mine, the choices were rocky and unsettled, unbearable. Even the women who wanted abortion unequivocally—a child she couldn't afford, evidence of an affair, misgivings on motherhood—even those women stumbled through the decision-making process, the force of the mind clashing with the body's poetry. I began to marvel at how women made lives for themselves, how we needed our bodies to tell our stories. How our bodies were our stories.

Ten weeks pregnant, I felt a change against my skin, something wet. I got up from where I was reading before dinner and went into the bathroom and closed the door although I was alone in the house. I was hoping it would be something else, but it wasn't. Blood. I called my doctor, who let me describe its fierce electric quality. "Meet me at my office," he said. "We'll have a look." He sounded serene, and I tried to take comfort in that.

It was a Friday night, wet and wintry, the cars all driving in the opposite direction, heading to homes of piano lessons, a glass of wine, the smell of roasting chicken. Christopher met me in the parking lot. In the hallway of the medical building the doctor greeted us, unlocked his doors, and showed us into the exam room, flipping on the lights he needed, leaving the rest of the office dark. He began the ultrasound, and the three of us said nothing as he concentrated on finding the bright pulse of beating heart that did not show. Then a sturdy voice said, "It's dead, isn't it." The voice carried no inflection, no male or female tone. It was me, because I wanted to be in charge of this, somehow, before one of them told me.

"We call this a blighted ovum," he said. "You'll probably pass this on your own, or I can schedule you for a D and C." I didn't want another D and C, the same surgery as the abortion. My body deserved the natural chance to accommodate this "blight." This time I wouldn't override it with surgical impatience or what was best for the marriage.

I waited through the night, cramping, and throughout the next day, the word "blighted" knocking around in my head. I felt limp and angry. Miscarriage was the shadow to a brightly lit subject. People didn't like to talk about shadows. They liked to talk about hope, and the unraveled pregnancy had no language, wasn't suitable for discussion. With nothing except the wait to occupy us, Christopher and I went to a movie. Right away it was the wrong movie for me, harsh sounds, lurid colors. How handsome and foolish the leading man looked, how superb and invincible the woman. The cramps worsened, Christopher seeming smaller and unreal next to me as the physical thunder took over my belly. I went out into the empty lobby, the muffled stupor of the movie coming from behind the closed doors. In the ladies' room the sweat from pain prickled my face, and I drank warmish water from a paper cup. The mirror was spotted and dull. I pulled down my pants in a stall to look at the heavy blood, as rich as cream, like something that should be good. My eyes traced the jagged lines between the small tiles on the floor. Other women had come in here and sat in this stall to contemplate some turn in their lives. They had stared at this floor. Stop, stop, stop, I willed my body, and went back to my seat, the dead thing inside me dying more each minute, inviting the rest of me to die, too. Each cramp washed over me like a life lived and ended, lived and ended, over and over. "Please, let's leave," I whispered.

Christopher drove us to the ER, where the nurse slid her arm around my shoulder and walked me to a spot made private by a curtain. She sat me down and took vitals, then eased off my boots and left me to put on my gown. Christopher sat in a chair a few feet away, and I couldn't stand him watching me. The sight of him made me angry, and I wanted the nurse back. I needed a mother. The doctor came and ordered morphine. I thought, *I can't take that, I'm pregnant.* Then I was lifted up out of the awful loss by the sweetness of narcotic, embraced by the dull murmurings of the staff. Christopher stood by my head at that discreet distance men assume from the OB. I was dilated and swept clean. He told me later how funny I got, making loopy jokes and giggling. It unnerved him, the sudden switch in my mood.

"Give yourself a couple of healthy periods," the doctor told us as we left. "Then try again." Hope, I saw, was back with its pushy agenda and wouldn't allow me to spend one day talking about my miscarriage.

On the way home we stopped at a restaurant because I wanted a hamburger. The laminated menus had big photographs of the food, glistening fries and obscene-looking sundaes. A sprinkling of elderly people sat in pairs, drinking late-night coffee. We dropped into a booth, Christopher opposite me, a beseeching look on his face. The waitress came, and I looked at her for the story of everything she'd ever lost, but she held a pad and a ballpoint pen and watched out the window as she wrote down what we wanted. When she left, we sat in the silence, so late, so hollow.

I remembered a distant friend who had gone through a couple of miscarriages the year before. I called her, and she told me she'd had four more, six first trimesters in all, six times the exhaustion, dizzy head, and lassitude. Six times nothing. We talked for hours, tracing back over our losses. She knew. Standing in a video store a few days later, I couldn't make a choice. Why choose videos, why make beds or send letters or put on sunscreen? Voices pulsed and blared over by the cashier's counter—*Due back Monday, receipt's in the bag*—and everyone was busy with acts and plans that overlooked my miscarriage. I felt dismal with isolation. An acquaintance approached me and said she'd heard from a friend. She said, "I'm so sorry. We've all been there." We. Our world, our important world of unnameable injuries. She and I had never had much to say to each other, except for prickly social frivolities, but now she seemed essential, a compatriot. I let her hug me. In the years after that day, if I saw her crossing a street or waiting ahead of me in a line, it was like getting a glimpse of a favorite teacher or aunt.

That weekend Christopher and I went away, needing to escape the emotions that had the presence of ugly furniture in our house. Maybe elsewhere we'd talk or take a walk together. We couldn't afford much, and we stayed at an old hot-springs hotel in the cheapest room, over the kitchen fans. I cried in the bed, the over-bleached sheets rough against my skin. I cried and I cried. Christopher sat at the edge of the bed, watching. I hated him for having the sort of body that couldn't do anything. We didn't touch in the night. I woke up Sunday to a gray morning and the sharp sounds of children's voices over water. "Marco." "Polo." Call, answer, call, answer. Everything felt thin and tight. We decided to soak in the steaming water, something I couldn't have done a week earlier. Aware of my feet on the hallway carpets, I followed after the skinny children who moved much faster than we did.

We came home to the same rooms.

In the following weeks, my anger diminished, but I succumbed to a fever of grief. Nothing was worth doing, and the state of our life together collapsed. Privately, I worried that I'd brought on the miscarriage, that this was payback for choosing abortion, even though I knew this was irrational. I listed scientific data and statistics every day to girls and women anxious about future fertility, averred that abortion wouldn't make them sterile. "The uterus is amazingly resilient," I said, but my fertility was trapped in a medieval narrative of special charms and impossible bargains. I read stacks of literature on miscarriage, looking for tea-leaf certainty that I'd eventually carry to term. I thought the word "baby" a lot. The miscarriage wound together with the abortion, pregnancy being about loss now, only loss, a big setup and a giant fake. Wherever I went, women appeared around corners, led by their pregnant bellies. Women stood up from loading groceries into cars and were hugely pregnant or dripping with children, the reminder of something I was meant to be doing, something I had failed to do. And, of course, in the clinic where I worked everyone was pregnant, and not wanting to be. I made an appointment to see a therapist. On her voicemail I said I wanted to talk about miscarriage, but when I got there I couldn't stop talking about the abortion. They were twins, my two lost chances, their wretched history carved inside me.

Month one, month two. Walking around, monitoring my "healthy" periods, I felt like I was balancing uterus and cervix on a tray, as perilous as antique china, as near ruin as old glass. Christopher and I hardly spoke, because I couldn't think of anything to talk about besides pregnancy—getting, choosing, keeping, losing—and only women seemed to get it. Christopher wasn't counting cycle days or sensing ovulation twinges. I just wanted a donor by then, and he knew it. He didn't want to make love that way, but I didn't care what he wanted. A cruel force came over me, the bitter, selfish intent to make him give up something huge in himself as I had given up. I stayed late at the clinic, talking with the other counselors and nurses in the break room after hours. We could laugh about anything, about having our hearts broken. Then I'd go home for sex.

More than a decade later, two children later, I can barely remember my husband in those days. The people who mattered were me and my unfinished babies, and Christopher's experience of that time—Christopher's miscarriage—remains as exotic to me as a language in a different alphabet. When we conceived again my body carried through the next pregnancies without event, forgetting its own troubles. Gradually, I forgot the gut-punch impact of the loss and its brutal ache. Sadness faded. In the story of my marriage, my strength came back, we mended and became parents.

But back then. The long, cobbled road after the miscarriage. While I wasn't pregnant Christopher just seemed stupid, and I watched for him to make mistakes. His only one was in not being able to lose as much as I had, and I was mean and raw and didn't feel the generous arc of love, the wish to protect him. I wanted it to be him passing the clots threaded through with dead hope. He should feel it, instead of me. That way I could be the one sitting at the end of the bed, staring numb and helpless at the other grieving person, keeping something of myself intact.

Mother of Three, Two Children Short

Joyce Maynard

Twenty-eight years ago, when I was twenty-four, I found myself pregnant again at a time when the prospect of caring for a second child was neither sensible nor convenient. My daughter Audrey was not yet one year old. My artist husband was painting houses for a living, and I was trying to be a writer. We were living in a one-room loft with a shower in the kitchen. When Audrey needed a bath, I used the sink.

Still, I wanted to have that baby, and when my husband pretty well insisted that we couldn't, I was crushed, although— here is one of the many ways a twenty-four-year-old differs from a woman at the age I am now, fifty-two—I agreed to the abortion. It was, my husband reminded me, proof of the necessity for the procedure that we had to borrow money just to have it done.

From the moment I'd terminated that pregnancy (as the language has it; one of the ten thousand ways we have sanitized and distanced ourselves from the full emotional impact of abortion), I found myself obsessed with pregnancy. When the

date came on which I would have given birth, if I had chosen
differently, I fell into the deepest kind of mourning, and for
two years after that, studying my daughter (an only child, till
past her fourth birthday) I would periodically summon a phantom image of the younger sibling she was supposed to have
had, playing alongside her. Only he wasn't there.

Eventually, I had another baby, a son. And another after
that. Wonderful, perfect babies, who grew into amazing,
wonderful children. Fertility was never the problem for me. I
took for granted the ease with which I conceived and bore
babies, much in the way a rich woman might experience
walking into a department store and picking up an expensive
dress or a pair of shoes.

The hard thing for me was never the biology of the thing,
only the marriage that would support it. Back when I had
agreed to the abortion, I said it was because we didn't have
the money, but the truth ran deeper, and was more ominous
than that. We didn't have the love, I think. The mutual support, anyway. Though looking back at it now, it was specifi-
cally the insufficiency of those things that came to fuel my
passion for parenthood. I found in my children what I didn't
get from my partner. I'd guess the same was true for him.

And maybe because of the loneliness of that marriage—but
also, too, because from the moment I had that early abortion, I
had felt myself to be one child short—I remained obsessed
with the idea of having another baby. When I had one, I
wanted a second, and when the second came, I wanted a third.
After the third, I wanted a fourth. And every time, my husband and I argued about it. He must have carried justifiable

bitterness over the relentlessness of my pursuit of a child (and what it suggested about my inability to find what I needed with him alone). For my part, I felt a growing frustration, and then rage, at my inability to control something as basic as my own reproductive life. I'd never pretend for a second that the pain for me of not getting to have another child equaled what a woman must feel, with a willing partner at her side, who's actively trying, yet unable to conceive. But all we can ever fully know is our own brand of grief, maybe, and that was mine.

I was thirty-five when my marriage ended, and when it did, one of the hopes I allowed myself—in the midst of all the sorrow and regret of my failed marriage to my children's father—was that I might one day be able to have another child. All around me, women my age were expressing their gratitude and relief to have the childbearing years behind them, finally. But as for me, I felt no less longing for a baby, after three of them, than I had when I was twenty-two and had none. Only now there was another element to the longing that I had been too young to appreciate in those old days. I wanted not simply to hold a baby again, but to truly share the experience of raising her with my fellow parent.

I had a number of relationships during those years, and always, when I did, I'd find myself conjuring the picture of myself having a child with this man, or that one. Sometimes it was my inability to summon that picture that caused me to say good-bye to a man. Once, it was my own firm stand that I wanted another child that caused the man to say good-bye to me.

I was approaching age forty when I met Don, a lawyer, who had never married, never had a child. Unlike my ex-husband, or myself, he earned a very steady income and had things like health insurance, and the kind of car that isn't likely to require a call to the tow truck several times a year. It took me a few months of spending time with Don to get used to the idea that we could not only go out to a very expensive restaurant for dinner, but that when we did, I might order not only an entrée, but an appetizer as well. Also good wine.

He professed to love me, and I think he did. In my way, I loved him, too, though I continued to recognize an absence of a certain kind of passion I had felt as a young woman, and longed for still. I saw him as what my mother would have called "good husband material." Steady. Kind. Faithful. Someone who would be a wonderful and devoted father, probably.

And so, as the relationship progressed, I allowed myself to entertain, more than a little, the notion that I might one day marry this man, make a home with him. The passion that might have been lacking between the two of us would find, for its substitute, the thrill of having—this late in the game—one more baby (who knew? maybe even two) with a man for whom the whole thing would represent a wonderful new adventure.

And then something surprising happened. (Surprising, because I was using my diaphragm at the time, and carefully, too. Not to mention, I was pushing forty with a short stick.) I got pregnant.

Though well over a decade had passed since I'd last felt that particular set of small sensations, I remembered when I'd last encountered them, and I knew without taking the test what was indicated by that odd tightness in my uterus, the tenderness in my breasts, the feeling that at any moment of the day, I might just weep. (Seventeen years earlier, riding in a car with my husband, a Stevie Wonder song, "Isn't She Lovely?" had come on the radio. The song—written as a celebration of Stevie Wonder's first child—begins with the sound of a baby's cry, and when I heard it, I had started to cry, too, and then I'd turned to my husband and said, "I think I'm pregnant.")

Now, again, I knew it. And though I wasn't in love with the father of this particular fetus, as I had been in love with the father of my daughter, all those years before—and though I had known Don, at that point, only a few months, and had certainly not planned on a pregnancy—how I felt, when I recognized that I was pregnant, was much the way I had felt all those years before, when I found myself pregnant, a year after my daughter's birth. Bad timing. Not a good idea. And still, I could not contain my joy.

I thought my partner—a childless lawyer, age forty, and in love with me, he said—would be ecstatic when I told him the news. My anticipation of his excitement, in fact, contributed to the happiness I felt, myself, over this unlikely development. Imagine having a baby without talking the father into the idea first over the course of a hundred late-night fights.

Because he lived in Boston, a two-hour drive from my home in New Hampshire, and maintained such a busy schedule that I saw him only on weekends—and because the thought of holding on to this information five full days without sharing it was unimaginable—I called Don up to tell him. But when I delivered the news, I heard only a heavy silence on his end of the phone. A deep, anxious sigh. And then the words, "So . . . you'll be having an abortion?" He'd send me a check, he said.

Until that moment, the thought of not having this baby had truly never occurred to me. From the moment I'd undergone my abortion, all those years back, I'd said that as much as I believed in the right to choice, the choice to have an abortion was not one I would ever exercise again. Haunted as I'd been by the thought of the baby I didn't allow myself to bear when I was young, I saw this one as representing a wild and undeserved piece of good luck. I had learned, long ago, the unwisdom of believing there is such a thing as a sensible time to have a child, and the folly of supposing things will ever be the way we might choose. Having a baby is about diving into deep and uncharted waters, under the best of circumstances. Sensible or not, I'd been utterly prepared to take the risk this time, knowing the one thing that was not remotely uncertain: Whoever this baby turned out to be, I would love her. I remembered how, when I was pregnant with my second child, I had supposed I could never again love a child as much as I loved Audrey, and then who should come along but Charlie. I had two children then; I knew the love of a daughter and that of a son, but none of that prepared me for Willy, a boy totally unlike his brother, all new. So who might be next, whose absence from my life would one day be as unthinkable as the three to whom I had already given birth?

Now, though, listening to Don's lawyer voice coming to me from his high-rise office, a hundred miles south, my knees gave way and I sank to the bed. Hearing his list of concerns (that we should have planned things better; that people should be married before they conceive a child—not to mention, he was up for partner at his firm, and the next six months were likely to require even more total commitment to his job than usual), I found no trace of the excitement I'd been anticipating. Instead, I heard the long, slow sigh of a man I suddenly realized would never become my husband.

"You weren't thinking of having it, were you?" he asked.

"I don't know," I said, sighing myself.

I made the appointment the next day. The pregnancy was so new, I had to wait another ten days before I was far enough along to have it. I dragged myself through them, less because of my physical weariness (though as always, when I was newly pregnant, I felt instantly the need for daily naps) than because a bone-deep sadness had taken hold. And though I told myself I wasn't having this baby after all, I found myself turning down wine when it was offered to me at a dinner party one night, and placing my hand on my belly when I lay in my bed. I did not cry, though I longed to. Audrey was fourteen now. Charlie was ten. Willy was eight. They would know, even if I didn't say a word about it, that something was wrong. No doubt they did.

The day before I was scheduled for the abortion, I felt a sudden cramping. The feeling, though similar to what I had experienced now and then when having my period, was the first symptom not to match any of those I'd known in my previous pregnancies, and it intensified. Then there was blood in my underpants. Then more of it. I went to the bathroom, felt a cramp more severe than any of the others, and looked in the toilet to see a little clot of blood. I dipped my hand into the water and lifted out a clump of something. I figured I knew what it must be, and didn't want to flush. I carried it to my garden, and though the ground was frozen, dug a little hole, patted the earth over it, and—finally—allowed the tears to come. No need to keep my appointment for the abortion.

Not right away, but some months after that, the relationship with Don ended. My choice. I don't even remember what the event was that caused me to conclude the two of us had no future. But now, more than ten years later, I know it is his words to me, spoken that night when I told him about the pregnancy, that remind me why I could never be with him. No doubt his caution was a sensible thing, and certainly our parting would seem to confirm the wisdom of his position. And yet, I find myself thinking that a man who could have embraced that unlikely conception, at a less than perfect moment, might have been a man I would not have had to leave, one day.

I didn't know it at the time, but that was my last pregnancy. The fourth child I dreamed of—the one I might have given birth to with a partner who wanted her as much as I did—was never born.

I've heard women who have known miscarriage speak of the grief they've felt over not being able to share, with a friend, or a parent, the loss of something that never had been seen as real to begin with. How do you mourn a child not yet born, a being too small to have necessitated the purchase of maternity clothes, even? Someone who never had a name or a face?

For me, the impossibility of expression was even more

puzzling. How do you grieve over the evacuation of a fetus that—if you hadn't miscarried it—you would have aborted? I hesitate even to tell the story of my miscarriage to women who have known the far deeper grief of parenthood foreclosed, or never known at all, when mine concerns a kind of foreclosure that only substituted another form of the same.

Still, that is the thing about a miscarriage, I think. Or one of the things about a miscarriage, anyway: However it occurs, under whatever circumstances—even ones, like mine, that would seem the least painful, most very nearly convenient—it is a death, and nothing less. It leaves you one child short, once again. Which means, for me, that even as I enter into my fifties, with three healthy, loving children, moving themselves now toward the stage of parenthood, perhaps—and me, having at long last shifted my dreams of one more baby to those of grandchildren—I am not simply missing one child who never grew, but two of them. I always know how old they'd be. What I do not know is who I might have been, had I become their mother.

"I Went Out Full"

Emily Bazelon and Dahlia Lithwick

Authors' note: *In the fall of 2003, a few months after we met over e-mail (Emily was then writing occasional legal pieces for* Slate, *where Dahlia was her editor), Emily proposed writing a piece for* Slate *about miscarriage. We both realized—to our great shock—that we had been working together professionally through the previous year without knowing that we had each suffered miscarriages, each struggled to become pregnant again, and that we had both finally succeeded. Several heartfelt e-mails later, we decided to publish a dialogue about our shared experience. It was a difficult decision for two legal reporters to "go public" with this kind of secret. In hindsight, we think it has been one of the most important things we have done as journalists. Versions of this piece appeared in* Slate *as a series of letters written over a week in January 2003.*

Dear Dahlia,

In a conversation about pregnancy gone wrong, the most harrowing voices are those of women who have miscarried repeatedly or lost a baby at or near full term. I'm not one of them. I miscarried only once, ten months ago, when I lost a pregnancy at fourteen weeks, two years after giving birth to a healthy baby. And though at the time I had no way of knowing I'd get pregnant again quickly, I'm eight months along as I write to you. Still, when the anthropologist Linda Layne says of her own seven miscarriages, in her book *Motherhood Lost,* "I experienced these losses as an assault on my sense of self," I think that in some small way, I know what she's talking about. Did you feel something like that, too?

Some women who miscarry find out from cramping or bleeding; others say they feel a psychological connection snap. I thought everything was fine until my midwife couldn't detect a fetal heartbeat during a routine checkup and sent me for an ultrasound. I couldn't see the screen from where I lay, so I watched the technician while my husband gripped my ankle. I knew from her expression before she said a word. I asked to see the baby—I'm pretty sure I used that word, since to me that's what it was. The technician said gently that, well, there were two. In the space of a breath I'd gone from buoyantly carrying the beginnings of one child to heavily bearing the endings of twins.

Mis-carry: The word itself creeps with guilty error, as if you've carelessly dropped something you were meant to hold. Pregnancy comes with a list of dos and don'ts, and doctors and the women's health movement like to emphasize the responsibility we have for our bodies. So, when you miscarry, it's hard not to feel like you did something wrong. I couldn't quite believe my midwife when she said it wasn't my fault. I kept replaying what I'd said a week or two earlier when a friend asked me whether I might be carrying twins. "God, I hope not," I'd blurted, daunted enough by the challenge of caring for one new child. "What if they knew?" I whispered to my husband. "What if they felt like I didn't want them?" I know, I know, it's crazy. But it still troubles me.

When people tried to comfort me with some version of "It's all for the best," I wanted to scream. I knew that most miscarriages involve a chromosomal defect, but the statistics weren't me. I didn't want to hear that my babies were better off not having been born.

That said, talking to people has been the best tonic for me. I had spread the news that I was pregnant after passing the supposed twelve-week safety line, so I didn't have the option of keeping my loss to myself. That turned out to be a blessing. Other women who'd miscarried—friends, a former professor, my sister-in-law, my boss's wife—helped me take my grief seriously. As I unraveled—there was a long time when I didn't think about anything else—I held on to the idea that I was joining a sad but wise tribe.

Still, I don't mean to suggest that you have to go through this to get it. When the father of one of my son's friends ran across the street one morning to give me a hug, I felt like he understood exactly how I felt, even though (or because) his wife had just given birth to their second healthy child.

Which makes me wonder why the common assumption persists that it's better, or in better taste, to grieve for the loss of a pregnancy in private. I wonder if the politics of reproduction have made feminists lose sight of what should be just as important a concern—the effect a miscarriage has on many women's psyches. Pro-choice women have trained themselves to think that life begins at viability; when we miscarry, we're disturbed to find ourselves mourning a child rather than a mass of developing cells. Feminists are generally much more comfortable celebrating happy outcomes than they are grieving for a lost fetus, for fear of acknowledging its personhood. Between 20 and 25 percent of pregnancies end in miscarriage, 3 percent of them after sixteen weeks. That's a lot of awkward hush. Shouldn't we be talking openly about this much more often, so that we're better prepared for the grief when it hits us?

Yours,
Emily

Dear Emily,

The impulse I'm fighting is to commend you on your "bravery" in writing so personally about your loss—maybe because it would make me feel "brave," too, rather than merely exposed. Which goes directly to your point about miscarriage as something secret and shameful—something two magazine editors, and serious legal reporters, simply don't discuss in public. One of the most poignant moments in the book to which you refer, *Motherhood Lost,* is the author's chilling description of forcing herself to give a speech at a conference just as one of those seven miscarriages was actually in progress, "so my personal loss would not be compounded by a professional loss." It never occurred to me until I read this that my own act of filing a story a year ago last December—the very same day an ultrasound revealed, like yours, that my pregnancy was over, and in the hours before a harrowing D and C—was similarly an attempt to show my colleagues and myself that my professional life would not be compromised by a dead baby in my womb. I'd have taken the day off for a broken leg or bronchitis. But something about having a miscarriage made it imperative that I never break professional stride.

You are right to point out the Catch-22 in which feminists are caught by dehumanizing babies before viability. But let's put it into historical context. The universality of the taboo on discussing miscarriage—the fact that our grandmothers and great aunts never discussed theirs, either—suggests that the shame surrounding pregnancy loss predates even feminist politics. I think we all falter around miscarriage because society has no scripts for dealing with it, and never has. There are no rituals, no expectations, no Hallmark cards for miscarriage— as there are in abundance for illness, death, even the loss of a pet. For the lack of such scripts, women who miscarry endure most of it in silence and solitude. "My Own Private Elba," I called it, as I lay in bed after my D and C, wondering why I was being doubly punished: first by the death of this first baby we already loved so desperately, and then by all the friends and relatives working so hard to erase all traces of it. I think I agree with you that one needn't "go through this to get it." But I also suspect that, with a handful of shining exceptions, the people who best knew how to be with us through all this *had* endured it. They either had the scripts, or wrote new ones. They were the ones who drove for hundreds of miles and showed up at the door, even when there was nothing to say. They were the ones who called and listened, instead of providing the universally cheerless comfort that this is "just Mother Nature's way of rooting out the defective babies." Like you, that line offered me no solace. It just meant Mother Nature was a bitch.

I miscarried at twelve weeks in December of 2001, just after we'd announced the news to anything with a pulse on this planet. Like you, I couldn't help blaming myself. If the authors of *What to Expect When You're Expecting* inculcate any single conviction in the newly pregnant, it's that if you eat your two thousand servings of grains and bulgur and lentils and spinach each day, stuff like this won't happen. They never say that exactly, to be fair. But the implication of all this "be careful" advice is that the shocking risk of pregnancy loss can be controlled. And I think ours is a generation of women who are uniquely captive to the illusion of control: If you study for the test, you'll do well. If you take the Kaplan class, you'll get into the good schools. If you drink your V-8, the baby will be fine. That's how we run our whole lives. But pregnancy doesn't work that way. It just doesn't. And later, when it's not fine, you have two choices: Blame yourself, or lean hard on your spiritual life.

One of the things I wanted to ask you, was whether all the rhetoric and poems and drawings of angel babies in the handful of books about pregnancy loss was alienating to you? So many of the pregnancy-loss chat rooms (these rooms are virtually the only public forum for coping with miscarriage) are filled with women whose grief is expressed through images, symbols, and beliefs that I found quite foreign in the days after my own loss.

After the miscarriage I spent seven months in that liminal space that can only be described as "not-motherhood." I kept marking non-occasions: the baby's not-birthday, the start of my canceled maternity leave. Mostly, I was nearly debilitated by the number-one symptom of life after miscarriage: blinding jealousy of anyone pregnant, recently delivered, or who even appeared to be ovulating. (Don't ask how I thought I could tell who was ovulating. Miscarriage-related insanity is a terrifying thing.) A friend who'd miscarried years earlier warned me candidly that you really never are quite okay until you get pregnant again, and, at least in my case, she was right. Which probably answers your question about whether my sense of self was assaulted. My sense of self was flattened. I became unrecognizable to me.

As I write to you, my number-two baby is doing that garbage-can lid scene from *Stomp* against my rib cage. And I can't help but wonder: Could you and I have read these pregnancy loss books at all—could we have written even one line of this dialogue—if we hadn't managed to become pregnant again?

Yours,
Dahlia

Dear Dahlia,

No, I couldn't have written this dialogue if I wasn't pregnant again—not now or any time soon, anyway. Like you I spent months as an ovulation-obsessed wreck, mired in the self-absorbed muck that turns other people's good news into reason for tears. I know some women find it difficult when their husbands aren't as affected by a miscarriage as they are, but I was hugely grateful that mine remained his optimistic, even-keeled self. If we'd both been panicked by the passage of each unsuccessful month, our family would have gone into a tailspin.

My mantra for holding myself together—for trying to re-gain the illusion of control—was to set a time limit for all of this desperate trying. If I didn't get pregnant again within a year, I told myself, or if I had two more miscarriages, I was go-ing to think hard about stopping. I imagine that's the opposite of what a lot of women find comforting, and I'm sure that hav-ing one biological child made the idea of forgoing a second one easier, or even possible, to contemplate. But I thought a lot about two older women I know who went through hell to have their own babies and ended up adopting wonderful kids, and I decided that I wasn't going to spend years measuring my self-worth by the stick in a pregnancy test kit. I wanted to remem-ber that being a mother is about the many years of raising a child, not the nine months of feeling it grow inside you.

When I got pregnant again last summer, I tried for a few days to pretend that this time, I wouldn't fall in love with the baby until I knew we were in it for the long haul. Ha. I couldn't slog through nausea and exhaustion and take vita-mins and stop drinking wine and coffee while fooling myself into believing that I'd be just fine if the whole thing fell apart again. I wonder how you felt? I decided that being pregnant meant keeping two colliding realities in my heart and mind from week 1 to week 40: My baby needs me to take care of him and to anticipate his birth. My baby may not be born.

I'm convinced that glossing over that possibility is a bad idea. My first son was born with a serious case of pneumonia; within minutes a team of residents whisked him off to the Newborn Intensive Care Unit, put him under an oxygen mask, and strapped down his arms and legs so he wouldn't pull out his IV line. The neonatologist on duty told us that he might die. Nothing could have made that experience okay other than Eli's recovery, brought about by a week of antibiotics. But the utter lack of discussion of sick newborns or the NICU in the pregnancy books I'd read and the childbirth classes I'd taken made me feel like we'd entered some freakish and shameful parallel universe. Am I missing something, or is the one-note insistence on happy, healthy births wrongheaded?

Like you, I'm not into drawings of angel babies or poems about flowers and butterflies. But the chat rooms are full of them, I think, because of the cultural and ritual vacuum you identified. I'll confess to you that in the days after I miscarried, I worried over what had happened to my babies' souls— even though I couldn't tell you exactly what I think souls are. A good friend who miscarried twice told me that after a time, she took comfort in thinking about her unborn babies. Maybe they're benevolent beings who are out there somewhere, she said, tied to us if only in memory.

Yours,
Emily

Hi, Emily:

You are right in saying that reading the literature on pregnancy loss is a perverse but useful antidote to the sunny maternity industrial complex that is made of pregnancy, at least in this culture. It is truly breathtaking, when you sit down and think about it, how much American pregnancy is about consuming, shopping, gifting, and hoarding. Births and weddings are the only two occasions that quickly become more about the stuff than the event. And you can largely control the outcome of a wedding. With pregnancy, and with little warning, you can suddenly find yourself on a million mailing lists, receiving hundreds of online communications about all the clever tricks your fetus is performing at thirteen weeks, then fourteen weeks, and so on. Every little onesie for sale in cyberspace is flogged in your inbox. I remember having quite a struggle to get off some of those e-mail lists when it became evident that the tricks had suddenly stopped, at least in my house, and the little onesies wouldn't be necessary after all.

You talk about your innocence before your miscarriage and the fear that pervades this new pregnancy; the odd schism in preparing for this magical new life while fearing yet another hideous loss. I had exactly the same reaction: holding myself back from the second pregnancy for weeks and weeks, so I wouldn't be fooled again. I wrote letters to both my babies through each pregnancy. The first bunch is jolly and silly, the letters ending abruptly. The second is spare and fearful and cautious. I don't think you ever go back to innocence. There is one overwhelming theme surrounding conversations about pregnancy loss: irony. And irony works best in the face of innocence. Newly pregnant women are like lambs to the irony slaughterhouse. We have no defenses at all. And this innocence exists largely because of what you aptly characterize as the "one-note" insistence that births are happy, healthy, and always successful.

I think one place that this is particularly true is in hospitals. Because midwives and obstetricians and obstetric units represent the Disney World of the medical profession—all sunshine and hope and magic—they generally deal pretty poorly with pregnancy loss. Layne's pregnancy-loss book quotes someone as saying that "hospitals seem to have no physical or psychological space" for women who have lost babies, and describes a woman left alone for hours after such a loss, because she was suddenly neither a mother, nor a patient, but just kind of a big medical bummer. Allowing all the women who miscarry into the world of obstetrics is like letting Dracula into the Enchanted Castle.

Yet when I had to have our fetus surgically removed, the procedure was performed, astonishingly, in the same maternity ward I would otherwise have delivered in. We had to walk the same hallways, past a pair of laboring women eagerly pacing the halls with their husbands, and past the nursery window where all the beautiful newborns had been planted in their neat, squalling little rows. And Aaron, my husband, was at some point trapped on an elevator with a million balloons, a teddy bear, and a jubilant new daddy babbling on with excitement over his new son and breathlessly asking how *our* birth was going. Oh. And the nurse who jabbed at me over and over with an IV needle, in a fruitless attempt to find a vein? She wore a name tag that read "Hope."

Miscarriage is nothing if not a festival of ironies.

In all honesty, I'd have preferred to have that surgery in a hospital broom closet or the damned parking lot. In hindsight, it's unbelievable that *any* modern American hospital would not have a soothing, non-ironic place to minister to the thousands of pregnancies that end as mine did. I am blessed in that my obstetrician was—and is—as compassionate and caring about the lost baby as she is about the live one. But I get the strong sense that she does not represent the norm.

So what does this mean moving forward? Can we craft a set of prescriptions for feminists seeking to incorporate pregnancy loss into their agenda? I agree with you that there is an urgent need to tell newly pregnant women early and often that there are extremely high risks of losses, and to downplay the individualist, you-are-in-total-control tone of the pregnancy books and classes. We agree that we need better spaces than anonymous Internet chat rooms or support groups for women to cope. But let's also imagine that hospitals, which thoughtfully offer massages and hot tubs and music for the new mommies, could also provide spaces—both physical and psychological—for the almost-mommies as well.

Best,
Dahlia

Dahlia,

You're right—if patients ran the hospitals, D and Cs and all the other procedures that surround miscarriage and still-birth would take place as far from the maternity wing as possible. But it's the medical profession that's in charge. And from the point of view of many of its members (many as in not all—to the exceptional doctors and midwives and nurses out there, please know that we're rooting for you), pregnancy loss has two things going against it: boredom and mystery. The surgery that we experienced as shattering was ho-hum from the perspective of the doctors who performed it. At the same time, the reasons why we were lying on the table instead of ordering maternity clothes were out of their reach, in other than the most general terms. My husband said that getting a D and C was like going to an auto body shop—a matter of fixing a mechanical failure without getting into the details of what caused it. The day before, the obstetrician told us that most early pregnancy losses are the result of a genetic defect. (Sometimes the brakes just don't work right, ma'am.) When we asked if he was planning to do any tests to see if that was the case with this miscarriage, he looked surprised. One, two, even three miscarriages are no cause for concern, he told us. Go home. Don't worry.

That response may make perfect sense as a matter of allocating resources. Why should my health insurer have to spend money to uncover the cause of a minor medical event that in all likelihood will turn out to be a blip on my fertility screen? From the point of view of the doctor or the insurer, waiting out a cycle or two of loss is no big deal. But if you're the woman who has lost one or more pregnancies and is frantically wondering whether you're fated to become a "serial miscarrier" (another unfortunate, heart-sinking term), every piece of take-it-easy, wait-and-see advice is a torment.

I don't know enough about either the state of medical knowledge or the cost-benefit tradeoffs to defend or attack the current standard of care. But I suspect that the science of miscarriage and its cousin, infertility, isn't really a science at all. A friend whose sister has been trying to get pregnant for a year and a half recently told me that her sister had finally gotten a diagnosis that made her feel better because at least now what was happening to her had a name—"unexplained infertility." No irony intended. There's so much about reproduction that we still don't know or can't fix. And in the meantime, women on the receiving end of everything from "just keep trying" to IVF face months or years of uncertainty and heartache.

I guess I do have one small, unprofound suggestion. Until doctors have better scientific tools at their disposal, they should use the basic tool they do have: human kindness. Obstetricians and fertility specialists can offer the kind of emotional support that makes you feel like you're not coming off an assembly line—the kind that the midwives in my obstetrics practice gave me and that your doctor gave you. And they can do a better job of asking women what they want in terms of testing and treatment and of explaining why certain options aren't warranted, if, in their judgment, the timing or circumstances aren't right.

The rest of us can also try to pick up on the cues that women give when they've recently lost a pregnancy or suffered a fertility disappointment. I didn't equate my miscarriage with a death. The longing I felt for my not-to-be-born babies, however real, wasn't like missing someone I'd known and loved. But I really appreciated the cross-country call that I got from a rabbi in California I'd worked for years ago. He said he was sorry to hear about my loss and that he wanted me to know that there were Jewish texts—scant, but still—that I could draw on. The best one was from the Book of Ruth. "I went out full, but empty has God returned me," Naomi tells the women of Bethlehem when she returns to their city after a long absence. She's not talking about a miscarriage; she has lost her husband and two grown sons. But she could be, as Lois Dubin points out in a wonderful essay from the collection *Reading Ruth*, edited by Judith Kates and Gail Twersky Reimer.

In fact, the image of being "returned empty" speaks to a lot of life's worst moments, I think. It means beginning again the hard work of filling ourselves up, in whatever way we can. You and I are blessed to be filling again with babies. And despite our previous losses, with hope.

Dahlia, I wish for you all the joys of motherhood—the salt with the honey, the vinegar with the wine. Thank you for writing to me.

Yours,
Emily

Dear Emily,

I'd wanted to end this conversation on a hopeful note and your last entry had me simultaneously crying, smiling, and wolfing down a grotesquely large can of SpaghettiOs—Michelin-tire-flavored, I suspect. Another *not* Sarah Jessica Parker pregnancy moment . . .

One of the wisest things said to me about pregnancy loss also came from a rabbi; a dear family friend who phoned from Canada as soon as my father told him what had happened. He talked to me for a very long time about how this loss would change the way Aaron and I viewed fertility and pregnancy and children forever. He talked about a newfound reverence for birth that we would feel, and that has proved true. There isn't much of the levity and fearlessness left for us—the goofiness that marked our first pregnancy, when we discussed naming the baby after Homer Simpson. But that levity has been replaced by something very sweet and—as you put it—full. I don't feel entitled to this baby, but I do feel blessed by it on a daily, almost hourly basis.

Like you, I couldn't have managed without some very generous friends and family members who then got me through the hellish first weeks of this new pregnancy—when I needlessly put myself on bed rest and worried myself into hysterics, until we had to rent a home Doppler to listen for fetal heartbeats so I could sleep nights. That was another lesson for me: There is no reason to keep your pregnancy secret from those people who will be your best supports if something does go wrong. Telling no one for the statutory twelve weeks ensures only that you suffer alone. I've learned that telling the *right* people at four days makes even the worrying and the barfing and the crippling lack of control easier.

When we started this dialogue, I mentioned that the hardest thing for me to hear after my miscarriage was either: "It's better this way, you didn't want a handicapped baby," or "When does the doctor say you can try again?" Both of these comments tried to erase the existence of that first deep love; like trying to set a widower up on a foxy new blind date at his wife's funeral. I wanted to tell you what was said to me that most helped, perhaps in the hopes of contemplating some new way for people to talk about miscarriage, or maybe just to give the folks at Hallmark an idea for a new line of greeting cards.

In the days after my loss, my wonderful cousin called from Paris, just to tell me that she had dreamt that night of our baby; and that she was now certain that there had been some purpose to its short life. And my literary agent—from whom I just don't expect sentimentality—told me shortly after that this was one lucky little baby to have chosen us for parents, even for just a few weeks. I don't know why such comments healed us as much as they did. Maybe because, as you said, it spoke to the possibility of something eternal, of baby souls, or some purpose beyond what felt at the time to be simply pain without bottom. Maybe because it recognized that this was not just the loss of something potential, but the gain of something tangible and meaningful.

In the past three days, since this dialogue began appearing on *Slate*, I've received stunning numbers of e-mails from people—many of them only distant acquaintances—who have endured brutalizing infertility, or miscarriage, or infant losses. Some of them were even in the building at work on days when I'd lock myself in the bathroom to cry. I just never knew their stories, and they never knew mine. They are reminding me, as you have done, that the only thing more brutal than experiencing these secret hopes and deaths is experiencing them in solitude or in shame. Maybe someday science will find a way to control for the shocking one-in-five reality that is pregnancy loss. But until then, we can at least try to control for the ways in which we condemn tens of thousands of our sisters to grieve all alone.

I thank you so much, Emily, for your kind wishes. You know, better than I do thanks to Eli, that with the birth of a healthy baby comes a lifetime of yet more fear and worry—about electrical sockets and defective car seats and (heaven help us) those Sigma Chi keg sucks of 2020. Someone wrote to me in a letter yesterday that I have now slept my last peaceful night. Still, I wish you some small amount of peace and great buckets of unvarnished joy in the coming weeks and years. And I thank you for carving out, in this tiny corner of cyberspace, a place to share sad secrets.

Yours,
Dahlia

Pregnancy and Other Natural Disasters

Pam Houston

In February 1997, I discovered I was pregnant. The timing, I thought, couldn't have been better. I was thirty-five years old. I had a home base in a beautiful valley in the high country of Colorado, a loving partner, and my second book of fiction nearly ready to turn in. After almost twenty years of collecting passport stamps and bad relationships and a list of outdoor adventures so long it was getting hard to keep them separate in my memory, I believed I was ready to hang up my back-country skis and my whitewater rafts and my whole collection of Lonely Planet Travel Guides. I believed I was ready to excel at the mostly indoor sport of motherhood. I believed I was ready to grow up.

For the first few weeks of the pregnancy I was happy, or at least able to convince myself I was. But during the second month a depression settled in around me that by the third month had turned suicidal. My doctor said mood swings were common but I couldn't make him understand that I wasn't swinging. I was down in a hole so deep I couldn't get out of bed in the morning, and sometimes not even in the afternoon. I was in a place so dark that none of the things that usually heal me—the sight of the mountains outside my window, or Van Morrison's "Caravan," or even the stupid pet tricks of my Irish Wolfhound—could make me glad to be alive.

Things will improve in the second trimester, my friends told me, but I couldn't even see how to make it through the day. I woke up each morning more and more sure that my life was over, that I had been handed a death sentence, and that even if I somehow lived through the pregnancy, the delivery, and the first few years of motherhood, my life would be devoid, for all that time, of everything I loved: grueling Himalayan treks, frigid winter camping trips, and the class-five whitewater rivers, that for so many years had energized and defined me. And as shallow and selfish as that might sound to anyone who has given up or greatly modified an active outdoor life to have children, the truth is that I didn't know how to exist without looking toward the next adventure. Those days and nights spent risking life and limb on the ocean, in the mountains, and down the rivers had been the things that let me know I was alive for as long as I could remember, and without them I didn't know who I was.

If those worries weren't enough to make me feel as unmotherly and superficial and generally awful about myself as I ever had, there was also the fear of watching my body change into something I could neither count on nor recognize. *Nine months up*, the books said, *nine months down*, possibly more for women over thirty, and though weight gain during pregnancy is hardly something a healthy person should hold against herself, I did, and in a big way. *A fat girl is nothing but a fat girl*, my mother used to say as she squeezed herself into her girdle every morning, *no matter what else she accomplishes in her life*. Of all the misguided rules for living that my mother handed down to me, that is the one I think about most often, every time a bite of food leaves the fork and enters my mouth.

It wasn't just that my body was bigger than usual that scared me, but that it had become, almost overnight, completely useless as well. *Don't lift that*, is what I heard a hundred times a day from everyone around me, or *Don't push it*, every time I went out to hike or bike or ski. But I had always pushed it, and I didn't know how not to. I shoveled a few inches of snow out of my driveway at five weeks, bled all weekend and very nearly miscarried, and the doctor gave me such a lecture I was afraid to do anything after that. (I didn't even tell him that it was twenty-four inches of snow and that my driveway is a half a mile long.) The challenge seemed to be to give up my strength and fitness for the better part of two years without drowning in self-hatred, and it was quickly becoming clear that I wasn't up to the task.

I understand now that much of what I was feeling in those early months of pregnancy was out of my control, a psychologically recognizable condition caused by a combination of hormones that soared and plummeted far more than they should have in what doctors call a "normal" pregnancy, and an entire childhood's worth of my own repressed memories that were fighting their way to the surface of my consciousness trying to break through. I understand also, that to say my fear of pregnancy was about having to give up outdoor adventures in remote locations is exactly the same as saying I love the jagged edges of danger—the rapids at high water, the back of a young horse in an open pasture when he's in turbo-drive—because they make me feel excited and alive. Both statements are truths, but only partial ones. And the deeper truth behind them turns out to be the same.

I grew up in a house that was filled with anger and violence, so much violence that I was afraid nearly all of the time. The violence in my house was bred of resentment: my mother's resentment over sacrificing a promising acting career to get pregnant, my father's resentment over many things, including giving up his most-eligible-bachelor status to marry my mom. If we believe the theory—and I do—that we repeat our childhood traumas over and over as adults until we get them worked out, that is at least one explanation for why I keep finding myself in the middle of all those tornadoes and hypothermic three A.M.'s and all those near misses with grizzly bears. It also explains why I was so afraid to give them up.

The only other time I was pregnant, my mother had said, *You have a very special talent that sets you apart from most other women, and if you give it all up to have this baby you will become indistinguishable from every other woman on the face of the earth.* I didn't know exactly what she thought my talent was. If it was writing, surely having a baby wouldn't stop me from doing that. But the thing that seemed to set me apart from most people—even from most writers—is what I wrote about most often: trekking at 16,000 feet in Bhutan, where I thought I'd had a heart attack; guiding a wild sheep hunt in Alaska that ended when a mud slide took our tents and supplies and almost our pack mules into the Sagavarnitok River; rafting down the Colorado during the highest water recorded in a decade and flipping my raft in the rapid known as Satan's Gut.

Having a baby *would* have made it much harder to do those things, and if I didn't have those things to write about, would there have been anything else? I didn't know the answer, but the question terrified me enough to have an abortion, which I did in a clinic where I stared at a picture of a sailboat on the wall the whole time. Less than a year later, I was on a sailboat that looked just like it, fighting off Hurricane Gordon for two solid days in the middle of the Gulf Stream, ninety miles—but it may as well have been a thousand—off the Florida coast.

What I realize now, several years after my mother's death, is that when she gave me her advice she had been talking not about me but about herself, and all that she had given up to have me. The abortion stands in the regret category of my memory, although when I add up the adventures, emotional and physical, I've had since then, they make a pretty good case for a decision that may have been arrived at poorly, but turned out, in the end, all right. And the reason I seek out adventures that come equipped with their own natural disasters turns out to be the same reason I was so afraid to have a baby. There is only one story of our lives and we tell it over and over again, in a thousand different disguises, whether we know it or not.

In late April, two months after I discovered I was pregnant, I had a miscarriage, and though part of my experience was sadness and loss, my overwhelming emotion was relief, like I had been given some kind of reprieve to figure out the answers to all the questions the pregnancy raised. Can I alter my definition of adventure to include sports that are several steps removed from real danger? Can I give my body eighteen months to be heavy and out of shape without dissolving in self-loathing and disgust? Will motherhood turn out to be an even more satisfying adventure than the ones I've had so far? Will I be able to work with my own childhood memories thoroughly enough to break the chain of violence and resentment that was so much a part of my past? Is it possible that in spite of (or because of) everything I've said here, the undeniable truth about me is that I can't now and will never be able to resist the sharp teeth of adventure?

What I can say with confidence is that I'm working on the answers, and will continue to, whether or not I decide to get pregnant again. In the meantime, I'm lining up a few more adventures. I'm going in December to ride with the gauchos in Patagonia. I'm thinking about another early-spring dogsledding trip on Alaska's north slope. I hike in the mountains near my house every day, and try to come down before the afternoon lightning starts to crackle above me and raise the hair off the back of my neck, before it slams into the tundra only a few feet away from me and makes me run as if from

God himself. I don't always make it below tree line before the real trouble starts, but I'm getting better at anticipating the oncoming storm. I hear it telling me in advance to take care and take cover, and more and more often these days I do.

Postscript: Five Years Later

I am forty-three years old. Old enough so that people have almost stopped asking me when and if I am going to have children. As it turned out, I did let adventure take over my last several childbearing years, but they weren't always made of wilderness and adrenaline sports. I was asked to take over the Creative Writing Program at the University of California at Davis, and I surprised myself by saying yes. When people ask me where my adventures have taken me lately, I say that I have been in the foreign country of Academic Administration, where I don't understand the customs and I don't speak the language, but I've found that if I smile a lot and show gratitude, the locals treat me pretty well. I am learning to co-operate at Davis. I am learning the patience it takes to see a collaborative project through. I have adventured deep into the territory of loving a child completely, though it is not a child I gave birth to. My brilliant and beautiful goddaughter Sarah turns fourteen this year, and we have begun to travel together; we have begun to forge the kind of relationship that lasts an entire life. I am dedicated to my graduate students as teacher and mentor. I am still capable of picking up and going to Mongolia at the drop of a hat.

There is a part of me that keeps waiting for the day when I throw myself to the ground sobbing that I missed my chance at having children. There is another, far more rational part of me that understands that I have simply traded one very valuable set of life experiences for a different set, that are probably equally valuable, and regardless of their value, they make up the path I am walking this time around.

PART II

In the Thick of It

Miscarried

Jessica Berger Gross

My husband and I had been trying for months. It was our second year in Los Angeles. Neil had a job teaching sociology at the University of Southern California; I was writing and teaching yoga on the side. We'd been married for a year and a half, and had big plans for the future—the books we'd write, the places we'd live, and most of all, the child we'd soon have. But things on the pregnancy front were moving ahead more slowly than we'd hoped. Our friends, it seemed, just needed to throw away their birth control for a night or two in order to get pregnant. For us it took boxes of ovulation kits, months of charting my temperature and cervical fluids, and prayer.

"Fuck," I'd mutter when I saw the faint pinkish-brown color of blood mixed with urine that stained the toilet paper. Our bathroom, tucked behind my study, was tiny and makeshift, as was the rest of the guest house we rented from our resident Jewish–Hare Krishna landlord in the almost embarrassingly new age hamlet of Topanga Canyon.

"Is everything okay in there?" Neil called.

"I'm fine," I answered.

I just wanted to be left alone. Another month of hope down the drain.

I was only thirty-one. And my menstrual cycle had always worked with clocklike precision. I wondered, more than once, whether this was the price I had to pay for my just about perfect, sweet and companionable husband. Maybe I wasn't meant to have it all. Or maybe thirty-one in baby-birthing years was middle aged, practically over the hill. Everyone—friends, Neil, our internist, and those hateful pregnancy books—assured me that it would happen soon enough. Be patient, they said. But after months of trying, I'd become a pessimist.

I admit it. There were many parts of my motherhood dream that were selfish, parts that were for me *alone*. I checked ovulation sticks and pregnancy pee tests like I checked my e-mail for news about my writing career. Two years earlier, I had left New York City and quit a research position at NYU to write, immerse myself in L.A.'s yoga community, and pursue the intangible work of "finding myself." In the time since, I'd written a memoir about child abuse and recovery, and was hearing back from my literary agent a steady stream of hopeful but ultimately disappointing news from publishing houses. Meanwhile I'd begun work on a novel, and was overwhelmed by the vastness of the endeavor. How much longer could I continue not bringing in a real income? Neil was my biggest fan and urged me—daily—to keep writing, but I was worried that eventually his generosity and patience would start wearing thin. I imagined that caring for our child would be the perfect complement to my writing, and the one and only way I could pay Neil back for all he'd given me.

I knew it was wrong to put so much stock in having a baby, but I couldn't help myself. I fantasized about knitting baby scarves and making fresh-baked bread, about having some reason beyond myself to get up in the morning and put the kettle on. I imagined growing my belly big, and eating plates of guiltless pasta. Wearing peasant blouses and stretchy leggings and clogs, with my hair plaited in a long braid down my back. I thought good thoughts about baby boys and girls and birthday parties and bassinets and flowered French cotton onesies and full breasts and, later, down the line, carpools and rehearsals and soccer.

And then, each month, my period.

The truth was I'd wanted a baby ever since I was a little girl. I wanted to love unconditionally, in a way that I was never loved.

I'd had a bad childhood, most of it unfolding in a rambling Tudor-style house on Long Island. My father belittled me, and hit me, and sometimes he hit my mother, too. Yet, inexplicably, many more times, he was exactly the sort of emotionally available father my friends longed for—he'd listen to my critical analysis of suburban life, drive me to play rehearsals and drama class, help me shop for winter coats and ballet slippers, and take care of me when I was sick, bringing me take-out wonton soup and cough drops and moving the spare television from my parents' bedroom to mine. When I woke up each morning I could never predict which father was lurking downstairs, making instant coffee and listening to National Public Radio or Don Imus, shuffling and refolding the *New York Times* over his cereal.

In front of me and my two older brothers, my mother always defended my father. I was a difficult child, she said. I had it coming. But in private, she sat in the upstairs bathroom and cried. Sometimes I would catch her.

In my twenties, my parents and I continued to clash. I begged them to come clean about the earlier years of violence, which they did their best to deflate and deny. There were years of therapy for me. And then, finally, admissions. A few months after meeting Neil, I'd gone to New York City for a series of job interviews and stopped home for a weekend visit. My father got mad at me for accidentally banging the stainless-steel refrigerator door against the clean wood of his new kitchen cabinets. He started turning red and yelling and slamming doors. This time I wouldn't have it. I railed at him for all he had ever done to me while my mother sat wide-eyed and worried. My father could apologize, he said, but he couldn't change, not at this late date. He was who he was. My mother wept uncontrollably. Although she'd been wrong to stay with him back then, she said, there didn't seem to be much point in leaving him now.

I stopped speaking to both of them that day. At the time I didn't know it would be a permanent break, but excising them from my life had a surprisingly salutary effect on my mental health. I didn't invite them to my wedding two years later, or accept their phone calls or letters or birthday cards filled with rationalizations and regret. I was done trying.

Neil was on his own, too. He was an only child whose mother had died of cancer while he was in college, and whose father died of heart failure just a few weeks after we started dating. His sudden loss brought us closer and that, coupled with my having cut off ties with my parents, made me rush the tempo of our relationship.

We fell in love in Madison, Wisconsin, where we'd met in a graduate seminar on ethnography and social change. Neil wore jeans and hiking boots and flannel shirts, and carried tattered, heavily annotated paperback copies of the assigned books. On our first date, he took me sledding.

This was a love that felt good. So good that, within weeks, I mentioned how much I wanted children. I wasn't exactly set up to be a mom at the time. I was living in a hippie housing cooperative filled with young students and activists. I was just about finished with graduate school, but was unsure where to go next—back East? Or maybe out West? Before coming to Madison to study public policy, I'd worked for activist and nonprofit community organizations. I'd wanted to save the world, even if I couldn't save myself. But now I wasn't sure what I wanted to do career-wise. I lacked a passion for my work. So there was nothing to anchor me to a place or lifestyle except my dream of having a man and a baby and a cozy house filled with love. All the men I'd ever met I'd looked to for answers, sizing up their potential as husbands and fathers and providers and lovers and magicians who'd make me whole and okay again.

Neil must have sensed my need. After a few idyllic weeks of romantic home-cooked dinners with music and wine and up-all-night kisses (and, later, breakfast, too), he suddenly cooled. We were sitting on rickety stools at a smoky dive bar on Madison's east side when I pulled myself close to him, and, drunk on new love, fantasized aloud about our future. Before I could bite my tongue, I'd started talking baby names. Neil's face fell flat. I was going way too fast, he said.

Neil was freaked out by the thought of having a family and the kind of commitment that parenthood requires. He was twenty-seven, still a student, and not even sure that he ever wanted to have children, much less talk baby names with his girlfriend of six weeks. He simply wanted to concentrate on finishing his dissertation and landing a job as an assistant professor somewhere.

Eventually, as we grew closer, our desires and dreams merged. We moved in together, moved across the country for each other (twice) and married. By our second year in Los Angeles, all of that "finding myself " had started to pay off. I rediscovered my love for the one thing that had brought me comfort and escape while I was growing up—books and stories. I began writing about my childhood, and as I wrote, I started to come to terms with my family history.

Meanwhile, babies became more important to Neil, who was finding that the more he embraced love—for me, his friends, even for the landlord's dogs—the more alive he felt. Having a child wouldn't take away from his life, he realized. It would become his life.

Finally, it happened. We conceived on Yom Kippur, I think. I had struggled since meeting Neil to find a way that we could come together in our Judaism. Mine was a mixture of the strict, rule-based conservative teachings of my childhood synagogue, and the pure joy I felt when I stumbled upon my own connection to God as a twenty-one-year-old trekking through Nepal and hitchhiking through Israel. Neil had been raised an atheist by Jewish intellectual parents in Berkeley. They embraced California and Christmas trees and armchair socialism. Neil and I found common spiritual ground in the Eastern philosophies that we'd encountered through yoga and the occasional meditation sitting. That Yom Kippur had been the first to make sense to us as a couple. The Zen Center of Los Angeles hosted services in their Korea Town garden, conducted by a California-style rabbi complete with gray-haired ponytail and guitar pick, who led services filled with meditation and song. We went to hear the searching *Kol Nidre* prayer sung on Sunday night and skipped out of the Monday morning service to do our private holy work. We were up in our tiny loft bed and afterward I held my legs straight up to the ceiling, willing a conception to take place. Later that day, I wore cowboy boots and a long black velvet skirt to afternoon services and we broke the fast together at a Jewish delicatessen in Santa Monica. I hoped that the following year we'd be coming to services with our child.

A week later, what I thought was my period came early,

lighter in flow and darker in color than usual. I tried for once to keep my sadness about our failed attempt from Neil, who had just arrived in Cambridge, Massachusetts, for what was sure to be one of the biggest moments of his career—a "job talk"—the lecture academics give as part of the job-interviewing process—at Harvard.

I pushed my sadness aside and cheered him on. There would be more chances, and new cycles. Neil did well on his interview and came home energized and relieved. But I wasn't feeling quite right. My period had been abnormally light and short-lived, and I had felt light-headed and warm that week. Friday night, while I was asleep, my brain put two and two together. The next morning, I woke up early and took a pregnancy test while Neil dozed. I looked at the two pink lines in shock. Crying with happiness, I kissed Neil awake. He went to the store and brought back two more tests. Four more pink lines. That weekend, after meeting friends for dinner, I felt a profound wave of nausea hit me. This was real. I was finally pregnant.

It felt like a blessing, like the best possible kind of reward. What happened with my writing didn't matter, what happened with Neil's job interview didn't matter. We were having a baby.

I ate whatever I wanted for the first time in years. Pizza and endless slices of whole grain toast slathered with cream cheese. I'd tried so hard over the past few years to be skinny and perfect and different from my parents and brothers who ate and ate. But now I let even that fear go, and tried not to worry as my jeans and yoga pants became tight and started pulling at my thickening waist. I bought two pairs of velour drawstring sweatpants, size medium instead of small. I would be a luscious pregnant woman, I told myself, an earth mother.

In turn I stopped practicing the sweaty, intensely athletic yoga I usually studied and instead took up the more precise Iyengar style with teachers who gave me special instructions to protect myself and the baby. My writing habits changed, too. I was so nauseous and tired that after unsuccessfully trying to write for a few midday hours, I'd retreat to bed and watch *Oprah* and read novels. I napped. I didn't feel bad anymore about not having a "real" job. Just a few weeks pregnant but, still, I was a mother now. My therapist said she could tell right away. I looked different, at peace; there was a glow about me.

I read pregnancy books. I memorized the sections on month 2. I made a list of the books my child and I would eventually read together—*Anne of Green Gables, Charlotte's Web, A Tree Grows in Brooklyn*—novels I'd loved as a girl, and ones that had transported me. Neil and I talked about names constantly. We wanted something dignified, something charming, something almost French-sounding, like Simone or Claire or Claude.

But what if something went wrong? The night before the appointment with my new obstetrician, I couldn't sleep. What if. Neil was snoring. I woke him up, whispering.

"I'm scared."

"There's nothing to worry about," he said.

The doctor's office was almost an hour away, in Beverly Hills—only the best for our baby—but it was less intimidating than I'd imagined. There were two comfortable long couches and a set of chairs positioned around a huge coffee table stacked with pregnancy, parenting, and fashion magazines. The other pregnant ladies carried expensive leather purses and wore heels or sheepskin boots. I wore flip-flops and a shy smile.

I was eight weeks along. Neil and I were planning on celebrating at a splashy Asian-Californian lunch place in Beverly Hills. It would be a rare day out together. That fall Neil had been too busy to come up for air, between taking care of morning-sick me, teaching, continuing with his research, and traveling to interview at the five universities scattered across the country which were considering him for a position. With all his traveling, combined with how tired and nauseous I'd been, it would be a treat for me to be in something other than sweatpants and out on the town with him.

Our new obstetrician, Tony Chin, met us before I had the ultrasound. I started going through my list of good mom-to-be questions about the delivery, the pregnancy, his ideology. What was his opinion on natural childbirth? Did he see a place for a midwife or doula at my delivery? Was it okay for me to practice yoga during the first trimester? I had my notebook out and was ready for instructions on everything from my diet to what side of my body I should sleep on. But when the ultrasound screen switched on our conversation abruptly stopped. Where we'd expected to see a fetus, there was nothing but a perfectly round, completely empty, placental sac. Despite my morning sickness and swelling tummy, the fetus had stopped developing days or weeks earlier.

"I'm so sorry," said the doctor.

"Oh my God," said Neil.

I was shaking, in shock. I was sweating. The air around my ears had stopped working properly. Neil came toward me, wanting to hold me. This couldn't be happening. The what-if was real. I should never have hoped in the first place. I pushed Neil away. I put my clothes back on and made my way to the lab room where a nurse named Liz waited for me.

"Are you okay?" she asked.

I shrugged and pulled up the sleeve on my sweater, and registered the comfort of her breast against my arm as she leaned in to find a vein and draw some blood.

Neil drove me home. Our tiny house was all windows and wood beams. A worn ladder connected the sleeping loft to the rest of the living area. I climbed up into bed. He begged me to talk and tell him how I felt. I just wanted to watch television the way I would when I was a child and sick. That weekend there was a marathon of *The Bachelor* on cable. I watched every episode. I ate frozen pizza and thick organic potato chips even though in my heart I knew there was no reason to fatten up anymore. I watched MTV—*The Real World* Las Vegas. Everything was trash, and I wasn't me anymore. I couldn't connect with Neil. He could never understand what I was going through. Something in me was dead.

That weekend I waited for the results of my blood work, and returned to the doctor's office on Monday morning for a second ultrasound on the chance that there'd been some mistake. But there hadn't been. There was no baby in the sac. Still, we'd wait for the results of one last blood test. That was the worst part, the waiting. I returned home and collapsed into bed, sobbing and holding Neil's hand, drinking ginger ale and eating toast to counteract the continuing nausea of morning sickness—never pleasant but now too much to bear. Dr. Chin called the following morning. My hormone levels were way down. I would lose the remains of the pregnancy but it might take weeks. If I preferred, I could come in for a D and C.

If, months before, I'd been asked what I might hypothetically do in that situation, I'd have said that of course I'd take the "natural" route. I was, after all, an organic-eating, yoga-teaching, Birkenstock-wearing granola girl. I hated even going to the doctor. But this time natural wasn't what I wanted. I just wanted it all to be over. I couldn't stand another minute, much less a day or week of feeling pregnant when there was no baby. Neil and Dr. Chin said it was okay, that we should do whatever I wanted, that given his up-to-date instruments the procedure wouldn't do any damage to my chances of having a healthy baby in the future.

A few days later, I went in for the D and C. It was afternoon, and the office was blessedly empty except for us. Dr. Chin spoke softly, he was warm and gentle, with shiny black hair and kind eyes. Before the surgery, he had me do one last vaginal ultrasound. I couldn't bear to see the image again, but I couldn't stop myself from checking the monitor either. Again, a third time, I saw the perfectly empty sac. We were led to a different room on the other side of the office where the procedure would take place. Putting my feet up into the cold stirrups, it was all I could do to hold my arm out for a shot of Valium and wordlessly make note of the vacuum-like device that would take from me the last of my pregnancy. Liz asked if I took Valium regularly. Many of their patients do. This was L.A., after all. We joked about how silly life in Los Angeles could be. I tried to act like everything was okay. Afterward, I couldn't stop crying.

~

There was traffic on the ride home. It was November, a week before Thanksgiving, but it was hot, even in the late afternoon. We had taken my car and I'd never bothered to fix the air-conditioning. How I hated Los Angeles and Neil for moving us there. I wanted to be back on the East Coast. I wanted a mother. I wanted my life to stop feeling so temporary. I wanted to be home.

Things felt fuzzy from the Valium and the shock. I crawled back into bed with a heating pad and the remote control and I never wanted to come out. I wouldn't answer the phone that kept ringing, not even to talk to my closest friends, several of whom had been through miscarriages themselves. I didn't tell my pregnant friends about what had happened; I didn't want my bad luck to rub off on them. Neil offered to make all the necessary phone calls, but I didn't want him to. It would be too awful to listen in from upstairs. Instead, he sent e-mails to the rest of our friends to tell them what had happened.

The pregnancy books, still in a tall pile next to our bed, reported that one out of four pregnancies ends in miscarriage. But I kept picturing myself in that Beverly Hills waiting room, the only woman without a baby in her belly. I felt bitter and alone. I wondered why this had happened to me—what good had all those years of eating right and practicing yoga and coming to terms with my past done for me?

Neil was achingly good to me. He brought lukewarm natural soda to drink with a straw, the way I liked it. He walked me to the bathroom when I had to pee. He held me at night, half-asleep, when I woke him up crying. He bought me maxi pads and gossip magazines at the store, kept the house in fresh flowers, and drove an hour to pick up my favorite Chinese food.

And yet I continued to believe that Neil didn't understand. The baby had been inside me, if only for days or weeks, but Neil had been outside both of us. He hadn't even been around during most of the weeks I'd been pregnant, as those weeks had coincided with his job interviews. And then, a few days after the D and C, he left again, for an interview at the University of Texas. He had to go—I understood that. I wanted him to go. He could call me a million times a day, but it still felt wrong to be left alone in bed, hunched over and in pain. Not that it made much of a difference when he did come home. He slept at night, and hearing his sleepy breath while I lay awake just made everything worse.

I was suffering from a form of postpartum depression, the doctor said, a chemical reshuffling of hormones. I'd feel better soon. But after two weeks, I still felt dead. There were cramps and bleeding, and pain when I peed or moved my bowels. The emotional pain was the worst part. I turned ugly. I became jealous of my pregnant friends, and the ones with little babies. I was angry at the single ones, too, who thought

I was lucky merely to have a husband, and to be trying. And I was filled with guilt at the relief of no longer feeling nauseous all day.

I didn't know why I was having such a hard time of it. Miscarriage was normal, common. There hadn't even been an actual fetus inside me for very long. The pregnancy books advised women to keep their pregnancy secret for the first three months. That way you wouldn't be embarrassed if things didn't work out. But I'd told my close friends right away. Now I felt superstitious, like I'd done something wrong, as if I really should be ashamed of having miscarried. Everyone said we'd try again and it would work out next time. Maybe it would. Months later, without meaning to hurt me, Neil suggested that the timing was better off this way since we'd be moving again at the end of the school year. That maybe this was God's plan, and that our baby was still waiting to be born. As if the death of this particular baby was nothing.

There was so much sadness that lingered during those first few weeks. And the deep disappointment of watching the cycle of my body prepare itself for a new life and then shut down for death. The lower-back pain that served as a constant reminder of what I had lost. There was the matter of the weight I'd gained. But while the pain of healing was physical, so too were many of the consolations. There were small tactile comforts in the most basic things, such as magazines and a cozy bed and flowered flannel pajamas. And then my first period after the D and C, the first I'd welcomed in many months. It came twenty-six days after the procedure, just as the doctor said it would. My body was beginning to return to normal.

I was ready to begin living again, too. Slowly I resumed writing and then, after a while, I went back to yoga class and even called a few friends. My girlhood friend Katherine said that she thought of her own miscarried baby as an angel, protecting her and her new six-month-old son. I held that image in my palm.

⌒

That Christmas, we went to Paris. It was my first time. We'd bought the tickets and planned the trip before I'd known I was pregnant, and though we were scheduled to leave only a few weeks after my D and C, I wasn't about to miss out on my first trip to Europe with Neil. We flew to London first and spent a few days there sightseeing and visiting with my college roommate who had moved to Britain a year before. On Christmas Eve, Neil and I took the train across the Channel. We settled into a small family-run hotel in the fifth arrondissement and began to walk around the chilly city each day, bathing in the stone beauty. Neil spoke French magnificently and guided me through his favorite streets, which he'd explored as a graduate student doing research at the Sorbonne. We kissed and held hands all day, and bought each other presents, and decorated our modest hotel room with red carnations and green holly. I pictured myself, a Jewish Parisian girl living in the early 1930s, smoking cigarettes and wearing lace-up ankle boots and woolen skirts that skimmed my calves.

I bought armloads of my favorite French notebooks, the colorful Clairefontaine brand that come in all shapes and sizes, and as I sat and sipped coffee and devoured the beauty of the city, I wrote in them feverishly. We'd had news, the week before leaving for Europe, that Neil had been offered several jobs, including the position at Harvard. My dream of moving back to the East Coast was coming true. There was so much, then, to be grateful for. We feted each other and ate simply and well—omelets and pastas and cappuccinos and baguettes and butter. We drank wine with dinner and came back to our room in the Latin Quarter drunk and ready to make love again. I felt young and pretty.

From the outside it might have looked as if we had the perfect life. And even from the inside, despite our recent loss, it was starting to feel that way, too. Sometimes I had to catch my breath and remember that this was real: my husband, soon to be a Harvard professor, and me a struggling writer with the time and means to make a go of it. In the romantic light of the Parisian cafés, even the miscarriage took on an almost rosy patina—it was an awful, unfortunate thing, but one that we'd pulled through together. In retrospect, there was only so much sadness I could bear. Our time in Paris was a necessary respite from the pain. Later, however, the pain would return. Back in California, after the arrival of yet another unwanted menstrual period, I would sob uncontrollably for days, feeling flooded again with waves of grief for the baby that by rights should have been mine. There was a very real little soul, I believed, that I'd lost the chance to know. Beyond that, the miscarriage stripped me of what even my father hadn't been able to—the belief that all you need is someone to love you, close friends to support you, and sustaining work. I had all that, but still it wasn't enough.

In the months that followed, I'd be shaken by the realization that the ways I had asked Neil to take care of me when I was reeling from the miscarriage were the same ways my father had taken care of me when I was hurt or sick as a child. I'd forgotten that, despite all the wrongs, my father had given me his love, too. Nor could I forget that after that first awful ultrasound, I'd longed for my mother. Or, perhaps, a mother I'd never had. I began to see what losing a child might have meant to her.

After my miscarriage, I tried to get pregnant again, with no success. I flirted with the idea of fertility treatments, but was reluctant to push my body into something it didn't want to do on its own. More and more, Neil and I came to feel that the pain of the miscarriage and our struggles with infertility were clues pointing us toward what we were meant to do all along. A year and a half after my miscarriage, we walked into a sunny social service agency in Boston and began collecting information about adoption. In a few months, we'll be traveling to India to meet and bring home our daughter.

During our time in Europe, I tried not to dwell on the miscarriage or other painful parts of my past. We stayed in Paris for two weeks and each day we spent there I grew a little stronger. On New Year's Day we heard a string octet play at Église St.-Germain-des-Prés. The musicians performed a "best of the classics" afternoon concert—Vivaldi and Mozart and Albinoni—meant for tourists like us. The familiar pieces brought me solace. I held Neil's hand and sat listening in the small wooden chairs of the medieval church decorated with centuries-old paintings of Jesus and strings of white Christmas lights. And I saw then that although death would always live inside of me, I was happier, most days, to keep it tucked away. Little by little, I could feel hope reenter my heart.

What I Wasn't Expecting

Jen Marshall

Ultrasound images can look a lot like television snow when the cable goes out. The technician's flat brown eyes squinted at the screen filled with a grainy, gray and white picture of my uterus and then she clicked the cursor on a black spot about the size of a dime. That, apparently, was our baby. All of the emotions I imagined I'd feel in this long-awaited moment, I felt. A helium-like mixture of love, wonder, and hope seemed to replace my breath and blood. What a high. I'll never forget it. I couldn't take my eyes off the screen. Neither could the technician. In an emotionless, too-loud voice, she announced, "It's really small. Measuring about four weeks when it should be six and a half." I didn't know enough then about early pregnancy to understand just how bleak that news was. I'd been too wrapped up in the getting pregnant part of things to think very much about what happened after the miraculously positive pregnancy test. A nurse was also in the exam room. She wasn't smiling anymore and her eyes were fixed intently on the screen. "What?" I asked her, "Is this bad? Should I be worried?" The nurse moved toward me and said gently, "Most likely, you do have reason to be concerned. I'm going to get the doctor and she'll explain what it looks like we see. You can get dressed." Then she and the ultrasound technician, who hadn't said another word, left the room. I laid on the exam table, tears sliding sideways down my face. I looked at my husband and neither of us knew what to say or do.

The doctor came in, holding the printout of the images. "Have you had any bleeding?" she asked. "No," I answered. Her expression remained professional and prepared, as if what she was about to tell us was as unremarkable as explaining why a knee aches. "What I think has happened is something called a 'missed abortion.' The embryo implanted and started to grow, but then stopped. At six and a half weeks, we should see at least a fetal pole and a yolk in the gestational sac, maybe even a heartbeat. But the sac we saw today is completely empty. This happens in nature more often than you might think. Your body should have expelled it by now. You'll probably start bleeding any day. If for some reason you don't, or you can't wait for a natural miscarriage, we can provide medical intervention." Miscarriage? How could I be sitting in an infertility clinic, having to hear that word after all of the other hard words I'd had to listen to in order to make it even this far? It wasn't fair. For the first time in my life, I wanted to destroy the room I was in. Upend the exam table, knock the specula and jars of cotton swabs to the floor, and, especially, tear into teeny-tiny pieces the calendar on the wall that illustrated the stages of pregnancy. Instead, I managed to politely ask the doctor what she meant by medical intervention.

"Well, we can schedule a surgical procedure called a D and C," she replied, "or we can prescribe a medication called Misoprostol that will make things resolve themselves 'naturally' a lot faster. That's probably the route we'd take first, as it is safer than a D and C. I know this is upsetting, but think of this: You got pregnant with your first attempt at in vitro fertilization. It'll probably work out for you eventually. Call us if you don't start bleeding in a week or two." Then the doctor rubbed my shoulder and left the room.

What I remember afterward was walking out of the clinic with Doug, through the waiting room filled with couples just like us hoping for some measure of good news—enough ovarian follicles produced, a uterine lining thick enough to nurture a pregnancy, a heartbeat. I envied them, because they, unlike us, still had a shot at that today. *Don't cry yet, don't cry yet, don't cry yet*, I repeated silently to myself, *try to look normal*. I didn't want them to know I'd failed the most important pregnancy test—the initial "positive" blood work and the congratulatory bright pink lines on the home pregnancy tests I took just for fun over the past two weeks meant nothing without a beating heart to back them up. Another part of me didn't want to scare anyone. I knew too well how worried many of the couples already were. Then we were at the elevators, waiting for the next one going to the parking garage. The tears in my eyes and the hideous feeling that I was going to simultaneously vomit and sob were getting harder to keep at bay. I stared at the heavy steel doors, watching the floors ping by, and wondered if I'd ever get pregnant again, and at what cost.

Lately it seemed like crying was all I did when confronted

with obstacles on the road to motherhood. But I wasn't always like that. I remember feeling annoyed rather than worried when I didn't get pregnant after our first few naïvely happy months of supposedly procreational sex. Few healthy thirty-year-olds think of infertility, after all. I had other things to fret about back then. Doug and I were newlyweds. And I had recently moved from my beloved Manhattan, where we could never have afforded an apartment with a second closet, let alone bedroom, to join him in a big, old house deep in the countryside of western Massachusetts where he worked as a financial officer for a small environmental engineering firm. Perfect for children, I thought as I explored the house's hidden staircase, charming nooks, and deliciously scary earthen basement. But was it perfect for me? What if I hated the long and boring country winters so much that nightly hot toddies became a necessity? After a few months of that, I'd end up a depressed, cold drunk. Not what I had in mind. I also worried that I'd constantly miss my friends and that I wouldn't find any new ones who would like the real me. I'd have to pretend to like ugly felt clogs and nasty herbal tea instead of high heels and high-octane coffee if I wanted my neighbors to talk to me. And what if I couldn't be great at my job any longer? I'd be telecommuting as a book publicist for a big New York publishing company, but neither I nor my boss had any idea if such a thing was actually possible to do well. Naturally I wondered who I would be if I ended up unemployed. And what kind of driver would I be after six heavenly, car-free years? I suspected that the old me, who I liked just fine, thank you very much, would necessarily change a bit with marriage and country life, but how much? And would I like the new me? This is what kept me up at night then, not the possibility that baby-making might be a little harder than anticipated or that it could break my heart.

As I soon learned, sometimes there's only a few months' difference between annoyance at not getting pregnant as planned and the beginning of going crazy. First I bought ovulation-predictor kits, which, if the smiling fat infant pictured on the box meant anything, appeared to be an obvious, neatly packaged solution to our problem. Month after month, the kits highlighted the forty-eight hours in my monthly cycle that were supposedly prime baby-making time. Still, we didn't conceive. Next I mastered the tedious business of charting my basal body temperature to even more precisely coordinate our efforts and track the results. Nothing. Time for more research. A friend told me that acupuncture could increase fertility. Although I hate needles, I signed on for weekly treatments and a regimen of Chinese herbs. Not quite the trick. So, on top of that, I gave up *all* caffeine, including chocolate and Excedrin. Alcohol also went bye-bye. Still no happy news at the end of my monthly cycles. Then I tried drinking gallons of grapefruit juice and green tea, taking cough medicine when I wasn't sick, and excising all sugar from my diet while drinking a flavorless, paste-like soy shake designed according to my blood type at the advice of a naturopathic physician. My skin and rear end looked fantastic, but I never got pregnant. And I was in an extremely bad mood. So I took the completely opposite tack.

We've all heard of couples who try and try for a baby

without success and then go on vacation or do some other joyful thing, finally relax, and magically get pregnant. Why couldn't that be us? I resolved to get happy. *Really* happy. I stopped acupuncture, poured myself several margaritas, re-embraced espresso and sugar, and told the naturopath exactly what I thought of her quacky blood-type diet. Doug and I went to concerts, out to dinner, on walks—things that had absolutely nothing to do with baby-making. And I felt terrific, like I'd been away for a month at an exclusive spa. And I *still* didn't get pregnant. That's when we knew it was time to seek expert medical help. What a relief it was to hand over the problem that had been plaguing us for more than a year to someone whose job it was to fix it.

At our first visit to the infertility clinic, the doctor, a plump, graying, glass bead–bedecked woman with a melodious voice that made her seem more like an artsy grandmother than a fertility specialist, enumerated the many ways conception can go awry. Hormone levels might affect egg quality and quantity or the thickness of the uterine lining. One or both fallopian tubes might be blocked. A cyst or other growth in the uterus could impede zygote implantation. Sperm counts might be low or the sperm itself may not swim well enough to reach the egg. As the doctor talked, I took notes and felt confident again about having a baby. There were tests for these problems and corresponding treatments, all of which spelled baby to me. I couldn't wait to get started. The doctor asked if we had any questions. "Yes," I said. "Do you think we will have a baby?" I already knew what her reply would be. Of course she was going to say yes. I tried to hide my smile. The doctor looked away and answered, "I don't know." She suddenly sounded less like a chatty grandmother and more like a remote and careful statistician. Then she gave us a pamphlet about the psychological services offered by the clinic and informed us that the therapist on staff also specialized in adoption procedures. Well, I told myself, she probably has to be cagey. Malpractice insurance and all. I stuffed the pamphlet I thought we wouldn't be needing into the bottom of my handbag and asked how quickly we could begin the diagnostic tests.

Excited and grateful as I was for the available tests, I also had to admit that they were hard work, time consuming, and a little embarrassing. Blood had to be drawn repeatedly and on specific days in my cycle. A miniature camera and dye solution were inserted into my uterus and fallopian tubes for a look around. My husband became familiar with the terms "collection receptacle" and "specimen." Still, I waited eagerly for the test results. With each "normal" result that we got, I felt a little thrill of achievement. It was nice to get some good news about parts of my body that I had thought were somehow damaged. But when the normal results kept coming and we were given the diagnosis of "unexplained infertility," I didn't know whether to be relieved or panicked. If the doctor doesn't know what's wrong, how can she formulate a treatment plan? On the other hand, maybe "unexplained infertility" meant that the problem was so minor that the easiest of fertility fixes, which amounted to little more than a few pills, would solve it.

We agreed to start by trying those pills—an ovulation-enhancing drug called Clomid—as well as artificial insemination to be certain the sperm got where it needed to go. I didn't get pregnant. So we tried the treatment again. And it failed again. I began to understand that the monthly cycle of hope and disappointment that I'd grown so familiar with while trying to conceive naturally was a thousand times worse when infertility treatments were added to the mix. We expect medicine to work. If you take Tylenol, your headache goes away. It was easy to believe in Clomid. I even browsed the baby clothes section at Target during that first go-round with fertility drugs, something I hadn't allowed myself to do for several months. So what if Clomid made me sweaty and mean-tempered for a few days? Who cared if the brightly lit, no-nonsense artificial insemination procedure reminded me of the "I Was Probed by Aliens" stories in grocery store tabloids? I could endure these indignities because we were making a baby at last. Except we weren't. Failing to conceive after having augmented our efforts with expert help let me see something I hadn't before—a glimpse down the horrid, dark well of hopelessness. Fear is a tireless motivator. I stopped wondering how some of the women in the online infertility support group I'd recently joined had found the stamina for six, eight, or twelve rounds of Clomid or other fertility drugs and inseminations. I also decided that we should move on to the big guns—in vitro—sooner rather than later, given the comparatively low success rates for artificial insemination and the way that panic and despair seemed to ratchet up a notch with each failed attempt. I wasn't in this to lose my mind.

Because in vitro results in pregnancy around 35 to 40

percent of the time (on average as of this writing), our hopes were very high. Those odds were far better than what we'd been dealing with. That knowledge made the daily hormone injections, frequent blood tests and ultrasounds to assess ovarian progress, outpatient surgery for the egg retrieval, and subsequent embryo transfer to my uterus much easier to endure. One thing I didn't realize before beginning IVF was how many things have to go right along the way. There is a chance that the ovaries might not respond to the stimulation drugs, that estrogen levels might get too high and cause serious complications, that once the eggs are retrieved they might not fertilize and begin forming embryos, that after the embryos form they might not live long enough or be healthy enough for the transfer. Simply making it to the day of transfer with a few viable embryos is a victory. When our first IVF procedure resulted in a positive pregnancy test, I felt like throwing the hugest party of my life complete with piñatas and a band.

⟜

Imagining a particular pain and actually experiencing it are, thankfully, two very different things. Miscarriage is something you hear about if you are a woman. What you think when you hear that word depends upon who you are and who you know. I never knew anyone who had lost a pregnancy (or talked about it, as it turned out), so miscarriage to me remained a vague, bad thing, a wrinkle in one's personal history that women had dealt with and, I thought, *simply gotten over* since the beginning of time. I certainly wasn't aware that miscarriage after a "successful" infertility treatment might be a circle of hell that Dante himself couldn't have conceived. The vast, blinding grief I felt when the doctor at the infertility clinic explained that we wouldn't be having a baby next October after all took me completely by surprise. I didn't know I had that many tears in me. Or that nightmares could be so vivid. In the days and weeks that followed, I dreamed repeatedly of a small, muck-covered coffin being raised from a pond by police officers. I stood by the shore, terrified. My baby, a little girl named Charlotte Jane, was in that coffin and I had come to say good-bye to her. Of course, my miscarriage happened much too early to know whether we would have had a daughter or son. But that fact didn't stop the dream from happening night after night. Another unsettling aspect of miscarriage was how fundamentally it changed the way I felt about my body. I had always thought of my body as a miraculously good thing, a vessel emphatically, joyously of life. I never considered that it was equally capable of holding death, except, quite naturally, one day my own. That sort of physical confidence sings with life so loudly that it's a hard shock to confront other, darker possibilities. In the time that passed between the terrible doctor's visit and the actual miscarriage, I felt like a coffin on legs.

As I waited to miscarry and worried that I'd never, ever be a mom, even just looking at a picture of a baby or talking about a baby was torture. Pregnant women on the street (and there are never so many as when you can't have a baby of your own) drove me to new lows of jealous despair. I didn't want to hear about or see any of that. Didn't everyone know how sad and frightened I was? Of course, many of my friends *did* understand, and I couldn't have done without their support. But nearly everyone else irritated the hell out of me, and sometimes for good reason. One friend actually showed up unannounced at my house, bearing ultrasound images of the healthy twins she was carrying. She said she hoped the images would "inspire" me. As she was quite far along in her pregnancy, the ultrasound showed two perfectly formed and growing babies curling sweetly into each other. Her ultrasound could not have been more unlike the devastating picture of my fading pregnancy I had seen barely a week ago. What was she thinking? Maybe the same thing that my mother was when she called to tell me that although I wasn't pregnant anymore *right now*, she still planned to continue acquiring items for the *Alice in Wonderland*–themed baby shower that she'd be throwing for me one day. Would I like to hear about the coordinating party napkin and figurine set she found online? Maybe after a few Xanax, I would. At the time, I thought that a person would have to be pretty obtuse not to see how devastated I was. Now, with a little distance, I realize that if I were in their shoes, maybe I wouldn't have understood exactly how much infertility and miscarriage hurts, either. Maybe I would have thought that seeing a pregnant woman would be a hopeful balm, evidence that wishes can be made flesh. Maybe I would have viewed carrying on with shower plans, in the face of undeniable evidence that such a party might never be held, as a statement of faith. I have to remember that I once thought of miscarriage as a "vague, bad thing" and as for infertility, well, I never thought it would happen to me and therefore, I never gave it much thought at all.

After almost two unbearable weeks of dodging well-meant sympathy bombs and dreading the miscarriage and yet hoping it would just happen already so I could begin to heal, I called my doctor to let her know I'd be coming in the following day to get a prescription for Misoprostol. I couldn't stand the deathwatch wait any longer. I also wanted to say something in person about the term she had used to describe my medical condition: "missed abortion." It really bothered me. The word abortion implies a choice. A missed abortion sounded like I meant to terminate the pregnancy, but then somehow forgot to keep the appointment. No description of my mental and physical state could have been further from the truth, or more insulting, even though I was, and remain, firmly pro-choice. I wanted a healthy pregnancy desperately, as do all women who make the decision to seek help at an infertility clinic. A search on the Internet revealed the term "missed abortion" to be an outdated name for an early pregnancy outcome better known these days as a blighted ovum. The technical definition for each was the same and basically what my doctor had already explained to me, but for obvious reasons I much preferred the modern medical language. I suspected that other women in my situation would, too.

I wish I could say that when I saw the doctor I communicated a friendly, clear-headed "just FYI" that inspired her to scrub the offending term from her vocabulary. But that's not what happened. As soon as I saw her, I broke down and begged for the drugs. I could hardly speak through my sobs.

My overwhelming impulse was to get the miscarriage over with, and she represented the fastest way of doing that. It wasn't until I got back to my car that I remembered I meant to tell her that the term "missed abortion" stinks.

The Misoprostol and the accompanying prescription narcotics did their jobs. The actual miscarriage was hard physically and much more gruesome than the "slightly heavier than normal period" blithely advertised by my doctor. But that didn't surprise me. Nothing about miscarriage had been easy—why should the event itself be any different? I awoke the next morning feeling a bit like Wile E. Coyote after one of his grand plans to catch the Road Runner had spectacularly backfired; the thousand-pound Acme anvil that always falls—*splat!*—on our canine friend instead is exactly what taking a dose of Misoprostol, topped off by a few painkillers, feels like the day after. But mercifully, another sensation was also present. Relief. I didn't have to wait for the ugly monster to show up anymore. It had, and I survived. Thoughts of what I might—should?—do in the weeks ahead jostled against the macabre ones I had grown accustomed to.

Over the past year I'd discovered that country life and I got along surprisingly well for the most part, and I didn't even have to retire my high heels. So maybe getting back to work on our crumbling old house, watching the garden for early snowdrops, and planning spring's first big picnic would make me feel better. And those things did help somewhat. The nightmares and grief receded, but neither went away. It turns out you can't shrug off loss like a scratchy old coat you're sick of, even if you really, really want to.

There are two things that I know for certain help to ease the lingering sadness after miscarriage. The most obvious is a child—your own, not someone else's brought by to "cheer you up." Easier said than done in some cases, of course. The other is friendship. Friendship can be the softest of sickbeds, the strongest medicine, the wisest council, and the change in the air that your heart will finally recognize as happiness returned.

One of the nicest things a friend did for me was to drop by a bag full of things that she knew made me smile—marshmallow candy, silly magazines, and bubble bath. Another friend sent a card with one of our favorite actresses striking a saucy pose on it. Enclosed was a flashy fake diamond initial bracelet—a big sparkly "J" dangling from a shiny silver chain. Just the sort of bauble we loved to shop for when we were single-girl roommates in Manhattan not so long ago. It reminded me of all the happy times we'd had together and of the fun that would surely come again just as soon as I was up to it. These friends and others listened when I needed to talk. They told me stories of their own lost pregnancies (one thing you find out after having a miscarriage is that you've joined a secret club of sorts) and I knew I wasn't alone. They went to the movies with me when I wanted to escape. They didn't let me hate myself when the inevitable and terrible feelings of jealousy arose toward other women with healthy pregnancies and babies. When it became clear that I needed, as the cliché so aptly goes, professional help, they referred me to a therapist who specializes in infertility and miscarriage. And they offered encouragement when I was ready to think about trying again for a child.

A few months after the miscarriage, my husband and I re-turned to the same infertility clinic to try getting pregnant with some of the "extra" embryos we'd frozen from our first IVF cycle. We were hopeful, but nervous. And rightly so. That attempt ended in an ectopic pregnancy, internal bleed-ing, and emergency surgery to save my life. I was devastated all over again, but not in exactly the same way. I felt mostly fear—fear that I'd never shake infertility, that I'd continue to lose pregnancies and go mad with grief, and that my efforts to have children might seriously injure me or worse. Despite all that, I had it in me to try one more time. That sounds more than a little insane, I know, but I wasn't ready to accept the possibility that infertility treatments might not work for us, and neither was Doug. We wanted to be parents more than anything else. My shrink said I'd know when enough was enough, when I couldn't face one more needle or test—that a feeling of certainty similar to peace would come over me. I didn't feel that way yet. Instead, I felt like an exhausted but determined mountain climber who thought she'd finally made it to the top, only to have the clouds clear and reveal a new slope rearing high with its peak just out of sight. I wasn't about to turn back. I had also started to collect information on adoptions both domestic and international. The file filled me with as much trepidation as it did hope. Adoptions cost a minimum of several thousand dollars and often many times that. I didn't know where we'd get the money. And the aver-age wait for a child was long—about two years, from what I read. Plus, adoption would mean really and truly starting over, with a whole new set of hopes raised and lost along the way. The thought of that made me tired in my bones. I'd already put almost two far from easy years into trying to get pregnant. If I was ever going to find the energy to wholeheartedly pursue adoption, I knew I couldn't be looking over my shoulder for the infertility treatment that might have succeeded.

Fortunately, I had a few functioning wits left as we sorted out our next step. I realized that I had viewed infertility services much like a shopping trip, but hadn't done nearly the homework I would have had I been buying a sofa. I expected to go to the nearest infertility clinic, pay the doctor, and take home a baby. But I never questioned how the clinics actually operated. What if some clinics were discount stores and others Neiman Marcus? We all know the old joke: What do you call the bottom half of the graduating class at medical school? Doctor. So I immersed myself in medical research, learned exactly which clinics were the very best and why, and we chose one—in Denver, Colorado, about fifteen hundred miles away—for our third and most likely final attempt. Our insurance covered only part of the cost and we don't have a lot of extra money. And I had to steel myself for the ever-present possibility of failure again.

The third time around was indeed the charm, at least for us. Shortly after beginning IVF treatment with the doctor in Denver, I became pregnant with twin boys. The first several weeks of the pregnancy passed without any cause for alarm, and Doug and I began, tentatively, to try on the names "Mom" and "Dad." All the same, we were also keenly aware of our luck, as we knew how precarious a pregnancy, especially for us, could be. And then familiar demons began haunting us.

At sixteen weeks my belly began to contract mightily, making even the simplest daily activities difficult. I knew these weren't the harmless "practice contractions" that happen much later in a normal pregnancy. My obstetrician back in Massachusetts sat me down to have the "if they come now there is nothing we can do" talk after he diagnosed the problem as preterm labor, not uncommon with a twin pregnancy. Was it simply impossible for me to stay pregnant? Would I never get to hold my babies? The vision of Doug and me one day holding our baby (or babies) was what had gotten me through the last two years. It was a holy grail of sorts. And now to be told it might not happen. That in its place might be a scene far more horrifying than any I'd encountered so far. Nevertheless, I made myself remember that these babies were still alive inside of me and that I was their mother. The worst hadn't happened and it very well might not. *No matter what, I am holding you now even if you can't see my face or feel my arms. I am holding you now*, I whispered to my boys, day and night, as a comfort to myself and to them.

Strict bed rest was prescribed for the remainder of my pregnancy. Friends and family worried that the enforced bed rest would drive Doug and me nuts—I'd be bored and he'd be overwhelmed—but we didn't mind. If staying in bed for a few months meant a chance at healthy babies, it was a small price to pay. How truly inconsequential, I wouldn't know until July 2, 2005, when our beautiful sons, John and Reid, were born at full term by Cesarean section. I hadn't even seen my babies yet—only heard their cries, because I was pinned down to the table while being sewn up—and already I knew that there was nothing, nothing I would not do for these two tiny boys. And that this day was not only the apex of happiness, but the beginning of a new life for all four of us as a family. I cried as I squeezed the hand of the person closest to me, the anesthesiologist, and said, "We've been waiting for this for a long time." And then Doug brought John and Reid to me and I held them in my arms.

Risky Business

Rebecca Johnson

When you are pregnant, you're constantly asked three questions. When are you due? What's the sex? Is this your first? I had no problem with the first two—I was having a boy, he was due in early September. It was the last question that always made me stumble. "I had a baby," I would sometimes say, "but he died." I preferred the truth to pretending that Luke had never been born or to resorting to the anodyne answer, "We lost him," as if he had wandered off at the mall. Nevertheless, I came to dread the reactions, the way someone's mouth would go slack in a funny way or their face would sink in an unfamiliar place, like an undercooked cake. Worse was the flicker of panic, as if my bad luck were catching. Usually, I'd look away, hoping the person would get the message: *I really don't want to talk about it.* However, that didn't always work. Once, I had to comfort a woman I barely knew when she burst into tears. Another, at a wedding, leaned in close, her eyes suddenly avid. "Really?" she said. "What happened?"

Fifteen weeks before Luke's due date, I began vomiting

nonstop. At first, I assumed it was the normal, hormonal scourge of pregnancy but after twelve hours, I became frightened enough to check myself into the emergency room where I was diagnosed with a severe case of a pregnancy-related disease called pre-eclampsia, a mysterious, little understood disease characterized by a sudden and dramatic increase in blood pressure that can lead to seizure, or even death. I vaguely remembered seeing the syndrome mentioned in the "complications" section of my pregnancy advice books but I hadn't bothered to pay it any attention. In my mind, sickness was something that happened to other people. Twenty-four hours later, my doctor recommended an immediate C-section. "It is," she told me, "the baby's best chance." According to the calculations of the sonographer at the hospital, Luke was expected to weigh somewhere around three pounds. When he was born, he weighed less than a pound and a half. Someone held him briefly in front of my face. I wanted to reach out and hold him but time was of the essence. He needed oxygen right away. The next thing I knew, he was gone, hooked up to a phalanx of machines at a hospital fifty miles away. After struggling to live for four days, he died in a plastic incubator, an oxygen tube taped to his nose. The official cause of death: non-oliguric hyperkalemia. Translation: kidney failure. I never did get to hold him.

Days can now pass when I don't think of him at all but in the weeks and months that immediately followed his death, he was my first thought upon waking and my last before going to sleep. I spent hours by his grave wondering how I was supposed to get on with the rest of my life. Advice for dealing with the grief poured in. Tequila was mentioned, as was therapy, church, a grief support group, and a Caribbean vacation. I tried them all. The internist who was treating my high blood pressure—a legacy from the pregnancy—wrote me a prescription for an antidepressant when I answered the question "How are you feeling?" honestly: "Terrible." I took one pill, developed a migraine headache, and threw the rest away. I wasn't depressed, I was sad. Anyway, how could a pill erase the images that were ruining my sleep—the panicky jack-knife of his body when he was wrested from the womb, the burned red of his skin in the intensive care unit and then, later, the purple hue of death?

The only advice that made any sense came from a friend whose twin boys had died ten years earlier after she had mysteriously gone into labor at twenty-six weeks.

"Have another baby," she said, "I never felt normal until I did."

Six months after Luke died, I told my husband I was ready to try again. For our "pre-conception" consultation, we went looking for a doctor who specialized in high-risk pregnancies, the new and unwelcome category we had now entered. From the wide-eyed way the first doctor we visited looked at me I could tell she had read the thick folder on her desk that carried my name and the story of Luke's brief life. Gently, as if extracting a piece of shrapnel from a fresh wound, she laid out the grim reality. If I chose to try another pregnancy, there was a 50 percent chance that I would develop pre-eclampsia again, and while studies were under way to find a cure—fish oil and vitamins C and E looked promising—there was no proven way to prevent a recurrence. I felt light-headed and disoriented at that moment, as if the ground underneath my feet had begun to shift. True, I had been in no particular hurry to get married or pregnant—I loved my writing career, and boyfriends for financially independent women were a dime a dozen—but all my life I had assumed that one day I'd put it all aside to become a mother. Was it possible that this would never happen?

"Many women in your position choose the route of surrogacy," the doctor said, as if reading my thoughts. My mind flashed on a headline I wrote when I was an editor at a woman's magazine in my early twenties, at the time surrogacy technology had first become widely available. Surrogacy, it had read, Womb for Went? Ha. Ha. I could afford to be glib back then, when my eggs and my life had seemed without limit. At thirty-seven, things were beginning to look a lot different. I may not have had most of the conditions that predispose a woman to pre-eclampsia—obesity, high blood pressure, an autoimmune disorder—but there was one I did—maternal age over thirty-five.

If that doctor seemed excessively empathetic, the next erred in the opposite direction. "So," she glared at me, "what brings you here?" I opened my mouth to answer but my throat tightened and nothing came out. I looked out the window of her office at a tugboat churning its way up the gray murk of the East River; if I could not tell my story without crying, maybe I wasn't ready after all. My husband explained what had happened and asked if there was anything we could do to prevent a recurrence. Watching her visibly relax, I realized why she had been so cold initially—she thought we'd come looking for evidence to sue.

Finally, I found the right doctor. Mary D'Alton, M.D., was intelligent, thoughtful, and chic, which shouldn't have influenced me but it did. A doctor who paid attention to what was current in fashion, I reasoned, might be expected to pay attention to what was current in medicine. It helped that she was a nationally renowned expert and chairman of the obstetrics department at Columbia Presbyterian, one of the finest hospitals in the country. D'Alton wanted me to take prenatal vitamins right away and a baby aspirin daily once I got pregnant. All the other remedies that had been recommended by various doctors along the way—heparin (a blood thinner), calcium, vitamins C and E—she dismissed, saying the evidence wasn't there.

Three weeks later, I took a home pregnancy test after my period was one day late. It was positive. When I had learned I was pregnant with Luke, I'd literally jumped up and down with joy. This time, I took a long walk in the yellow woods of autumn and had a cry. If this child died on me, as Luke had, I didn't know if I could take it. The previous year, my ninety-nine-year-old grandmother died at home in her bed; a few months later my father had a stroke and died at the hospital. I grieved for them both but the pain didn't compare with losing Luke. We learn, early in life, to accept the death of our elders. It's sad but it's life. My grandmother was old. My father had a bad heart and smoked two packs a day. In the natural order of the universe, their deaths made sense. When that order is reversed and a child dies, it's as if the world has come to an end.

It may even be that we let ourselves love our children as unconditionally as we do because we believe we won't have to watch them die. I don't think of myself as a brave person partly because I have been coddled by the conveniences of modern life and untested by the physical hardship that used to characterize the vast majority of life on the planet. If I had yearned for an opportunity to be tested (I hadn't, actually) here it was.

Six weeks later, I was back in Dr. D'Alton's office for a sonogram. Before Luke died, I used to look forward to the machine and the tantalizing puzzle of its snowy image—is that a foot or a head?—but ever since the last one, I had come to fear the machine and its ability to foretell disaster. Lying on the gurney, holding my husband's hand, I kept my eyes glued to the screen watching for the frantic pulse of an early heartbeat in the gray fuzz of the image. Nothing was moving.

"There's no heartbeat," I said.

"Yes, there is!" my husband answered, disbelieving. The young woman performing the test looked at me blankly and said she'd be right back. When Dr. D'Alton entered the room a few minutes later, her face grave, I knew.

It surprised me how little I grieved over that pregnancy. In the months after Luke died, other women had tried to empathize with me by offering up their own experiences with miscarriage. They meant well, but once I had been through both, I knew there was no comparison. At six weeks, there had been no body or face, no head with hair or feet with toes. I had not lived with the child for six months, growing accustomed to his periods of wakefulness and sleep. I had not given him a name or planned his future. I had not watched him lose the fight to live. One out of four pregnancies ends in miscarriage; this was simply nature's way of saying "Not this one, not yet." As a fertility doctor whom I interviewed once said to me, "Nature is extraordinarily wasteful when it comes to reproduction—look at all the acorns on the forest floor."

Two months later, one of those acorns sprouted and we got a heartbeat at six weeks. I was happy, but wary, and kept the news quiet, telling only family and close friends. I'd seen enough of pregnancy to understand that the road from a pink line on a plastic stick to a healthy baby is long, and far from simple. Around week seven, I began throwing up again. Before, I had viewed the unpleasant side effects of pregnancy—the nausea, the sleeplessness, the swelling—as necessary evils, part of the vast array of feminine complaints that begin with the pain of the first period and end with the hot flash of menopause. This time around, I viewed all those side effects not as points of reference for bonding with other soon-to-be mothers, but as potential symptoms of a deadly disease, something my new doctor, specializing in high-risk pregnancies, never let me forget.

"How are you?" Dr. D'Alton would ask on my weekly visits to her office. My last doctor had seen me only once every four weeks, standard care until the third trimester.

"Good," I'd answer, falsely chipper, trying to evade her searching gaze. Ours was a complicated relationship. On the one hand, I wanted her to be vigilant; perhaps if my last doctor had paid more attention to my symptoms, Luke might be alive. On the other hand, I was so desperate for the pregnancy to be normal, I was tempted to downplay my complaints, to not mention the lassitude and nausea that dogged me daily.

"You look tired," she'd say.

"I *am* tired," I'd answer, thinking she was being conversational.

"You shouldn't be," she'd reply, ordering a battery of tests, all of which consistently came back negative.

By the second trimester the nausea began to ease and I went back to work. One morning, having spent the previous evening at a party with an interview subject, I woke too exhausted to make my nine A.M. appointment. A few hours later, Dr. D'Alton called.

"Rebecca," she chastised me, "you have to make this pregnancy a priority."

I opened my mouth to defend myself but then bit my tongue. I was lucky to have a doctor who cared. Besides, how could she know that I thought of little else? Especially as we drew close to the twenty-five-week mark, the time when Luke had been born. By then, I could usually feel the new baby kick on a fairly regular basis, but sometimes I couldn't. On the days I couldn't, I became convinced the baby was sick or, worse, dead. One afternoon, my husband walked into our bedroom to find me listening to my swollen stomach with the stethoscope from the blood pressure monitor cuff we'd bought to measure my pressure at home.

"What are you doing?" he asked.

"Nothing," I answered, hiding the cuff under the covers. I was listening for the baby's heart, and I knew he wouldn't approve. He is a highly rational man. Taking the cuff away from me, he pointed out that I would need something a lot stronger to hear a baby's heartbeat—true, all I could hear was the bully thud of my own organ—and, by the way, if I continued this way I was going to make myself crazy. That afternoon, I found a company on the Internet that rented fetal heart-rate detectors for only twenty-eight dollars a month. "Listen to your baby's heart in the comfort of your own home!" the ad for the Doppler Dynamo read. I knew better than to mention it to my husband, but when I asked the midwife who checked my vital signs weekly what she thought about it, she also looked horrified.

"Absolutely not," she said, "you are going to make yourself crazy." I was, I noticed, beginning to hear the word "crazy" uttered more and more often.

Around week 28, the nausea returned, along with a nasty case of heartburn. In my mind, the two were linked but Dr. D'Alton suspected pre-eclampsia. Twice, she sent me to the hospital for observation. I'd spend the day in labor and delivery triage, hooked up to a fetal heart-rate monitor, watching as other women on the brink of delivery would arrive, doubled over in pain. The sounds of our baby's heartbeats filled the room, like the rhythmic thrum of a large aquarium, horses' hooves galloping in the distance. Each time, my lab results came back normal. As soon as I got the good news, I'd dress quickly and leave the hospital as fast as I could, vaguely sheepish for having taken a bed away from someone who actually needed it.

At thirty-four weeks, almost six weeks before he was technically due, Mary (as I now referred to Dr. D'Alton) decided it was time for me to deliver. I knew she thought the nausea was psychosomatic—"I'm not saying you're crazy," she once said, "but anxiety could be playing a role here"—but neither did she want to take a chance. I fretted for a day. Was the baby ready? Were we taking him too early? I had kicked myself many times over for being too passive in the debacle of my first pregnancy. I should have known more, I should have asked better questions, I shouldn't have acquiesced so easily. Was I making the same mistake? I called the doctor who had treated Luke in the neonatal intensive care unit, a wise man whose compassion had helped us enormously in those dark days. "There is," he reassured me, "no comparison between a baby born at Luke's age and one born at thirty-five weeks." I called Mary and gave her the go-ahead.

The day before the operation was scheduled, my mother arrived to help with the baby. "Where is everything?" she asked, perplexed, when I showed her the empty room that was going to be the nursery. How could I tell her that simply buying diapers spooked me? One of the few things I'd been grateful for after Luke's death was my procrastination in setting up his room. I knew how cruel fate could be, and I didn't want to tempt him. As if to prove me right, the afternoon before my surgery was scheduled the lights went out all over the Northeast. I couldn't get in touch with Mary or her office. As night fell, my husband and I sat in his car, listening to the news on the radio. A reporter announced that hospitals across the city were taking emergencies only. In the green glow of the radio's light, we debated whether my C-section could be considered an emergency and came to the reluctant conclusion that the answer was probably "no."

The next morning, the phone rang at 6:45 A.M. It was

the midwife from Mary's office. "Where are you?" she asked. We drove to the hospital at ninety miles an hour. If we got stopped, I figured we had the perfect excuse.

Four days later, my husband and I brought our new son, Simon Porter Smith, home from the hospital. He was a beautiful baby boy weighing six pounds, five ounces, with murky blue eyes, a healthy head of brown hair, and a perplexed expression on his face that seemed to ask "Why am I here?" When we passed the grocery store, I told my husband to pull over. We needed to buy diapers.

Unplanned

Jessica Jernigan

1.

I had not been trying to get pregnant.

I was washing the breakfast dishes one morning when it occurred to me that my breasts had been swollen and sore for a couple of weeks. This sometimes happens just before my period, but this time my period didn't seem to be coming. I considered this physiological oddity alongside a recent sexual indiscretion, and I knew that I was pregnant.

I had thought that I might be pregnant before—my period would be a few days late and I would start to worry that bad luck had finally prevailed over latex, spermicide, and the pill—but this was different. I was certain I was right, and, this time, I wasn't afraid.

I finished the dishes, dried my steady hands, and started making a grocery list. I was living in the mountains then, and it was winter. If I was making a trip into town for a home pregnancy test, I might as well pick up a few other things while I was out. I looked around the kitchen, and I thought about what I would be needing now: vitamins, leafy greens, some lean meat, a pound of decaf. I grabbed my coat, pulled on some boots, and headed for the store.

When I got back to the house, I put the groceries away and took the pregnancy test into the bathroom. I peed on the stick, set the test on the edge of the sink, and walked into the hallway to wait.

It was a sunny day, and cool light bounced off the snow, pouring through the windows. Everything sparkled. I have never felt so sure of myself, so knowing and so content, as I was at that moment. I had become a new person, one who was going to have a baby, who was going to be a mother. I felt like I had never been more truly myself. I was ecstatic.

I had always assumed that I would have kids someday, but motherhood had been an abstraction, an idea that belonged to an indefinite point in the future. There were times in the past when I really had not been ready, when I would have had an abortion if I had discovered that I was pregnant. But now, abortion didn't even occur to me. Motherhood was immediate and absolutely real, and I knew that I had never wanted anything more than I wanted to have this baby.

2.

I loved being pregnant. It was so easy to be good to myself when that meant being good to my baby. I had developed the wintertime ritual of settling in by the fireplace after dinner to sip cognac and have one cigarette while I read. I didn't even miss the booze or the smoke when pregnancy necessitated that I give them up. Contrary to a lifetime of overindulgence and indifference to nutrition, my diet became exemplary—full of vegetables and protein and healthy fats. I strapped on snowshoes every day for a gently invigorating stroll through the trees.

I loved myself while I was pregnant. My relationship with my body had always been ambivalent at best. Now, constantly aware and amazed that I had a child growing inside me, I was able to see myself as more than a generally unsatisfying reflection in the mirror. My flesh was—it was obvious to me now—a miracle. When I think back on this time, the image that comes to me most readily is my little bed in a cozy attic room, and me luxuriating in a nap while the afternoon sun flickered across the ceiling. I remember feeling utterly, perfectly fulfilled.

Carrying a child didn't merely alter my experience of my body. Carrying a child opened my eyes to a reality greater than myself. I had felt loved—honestly and deeply and unreservedly—before I got pregnant, but now I felt something more. I didn't just feel loved—I felt like I was *inside* love. I did not comprehend this feeling as God, but as Life. It was as if I looked around myself—outside myself, beyond myself—and said, "Ah, yes. *Now* I get it." I felt like I understood for the first time what people mean when they say they are blessed. Being pregnant was bliss, and I was so grateful for it and so amazed, because it was unsought and unplanned.

I had just turned thirty. I had a good job and a nice place to live. I felt absolutely ready to be a parent. The only doubt

I experienced, the only flicker of unease, was when I thought of my baby's father.

3.

"Who is *that?*"

This is what I asked my friend Anna the first time Luke walked past my cubicle.

"Oh my God: I know." This was Anna's response. We share a fondness for men whose undeniable good looks are offset by a pleasing geekiness. His brown hair was disheveled—not artfully, but honestly. He was skinny without being scrawny. He favored thrift-store sweaters. His eyes were blue.

Anna worked in the same office building as I did and, as it turned out, Luke was the new guy in her department. So, I had his name and his e-mail address, but no reason—besides a mildly feverish infatuation, which did not strike me as a cool opener—to get in touch.

He and I both lived in Ann Arbor, both of us close to downtown. It seemed like I started noticing him whenever I went out—in bookstores, coffee shops, or strolling around—and, after it was obvious that random encounters had turned into mutual recognition, I asked him out. He accepted.

We met at a nice bar downtown. We shared a bottle of Côtes du Rhône and we talked. We talked about science fiction and philosophy and music. Luke was obviously smart and awkwardly charming, full of delightfully oddball surprises. It was such a pleasure to know that I could make jokes about

Foucault or references to Asimov's laws of robotics without fear of being incomprehensible, and I believe I did a more than creditable job with my end of the conversation. Also, I was wearing a tight sweater, which I often find helpful in such situations.

After we finished our bottle of wine, we went for a walk that ended at my front door. As we were saying good night, I kissed Luke. He kissed me back. Then he asked me if I would like to go to his place, and it took exactly no deliberation on my part to determine that I would like that very much.

This was my first-ever attempt at casual sex; never before had I gone to bed with a man on the first date and, as it would soon be apparent, I'm not very good at casual sex. The sex was fine, but the casual part was beyond me. I was pretty much in love with Luke by the time we fell asleep.

4.

I got the first inkling that I was more into him than he was into me the following morning, as I was leaving his apartment. My kiss good-bye was a little more enthusiastic, and a lot more promising, than his. I convinced myself that he was just tired, and thus began our rather tortured relationship, the tone of our "romance" more or less foretold in that unfortunate morning-after kiss.

Luke and I spent a good deal of time together over the next several weeks. We went out for coffee, for drinks, for dinner. We attended a few parties together. We had sex. We looked like a couple—and I was certainly trying to act like part of a couple—but Luke was reserved. In fact, he was quite honest—gentle, even kind, but utterly forthright—about his failure to be in love with me. Sometimes, I would even try to listen to what he was saying, but, mostly, I believed that eventually he would discover what I already knew, that we were meant to be together. My strategy was to stick around until he came to his senses and loved me like I loved him.

Clearly, I was insane. There were moments of cold, cruel clarity in which I understood this—even then—but those moments were fleeting. On the whole, I persisted in my delusion, sometimes discouraged and sometimes encouraged by Luke. I spent a lot of time on the phone, analyzing his every word and deed while my friends listened. A couple of them hated him: They thought he was a dick, heartlessly using me for sex, and they had no tolerance for my attempts to defend him. Other friends agreed that, yes, he was crazy not to be in love with me, but everyone concurred that I should cut my losses and move on. Some of my friends expressed this judgment more gently than others, but it was—certainly—the consensus opinion.

It would have been much easier—not easy, but easier—to agree with them if Luke had, in fact, been an asshole. In some ways, Luke was self-centered, but this trait tended to manifest itself as a confused, sometimes misguided sort of selflessness. I think he continued to see me when a wiser man would have run screaming because he felt responsible for me. It's also true that we did have much in common, and that, when things weren't fraught and frantic, we enjoyed each other's company very much. We saw art-house movies together. We went to concerts. We continued to talk about books and ideas. Also, he seemed to appreciate the sex. I believe that we were both doing the best that we could in a hopeless but not altogether unpleasant situation. It's just that our best wasn't especially good.

This state of affairs might have endured indefinitely, if not for a friend who offered both her opinion that I should get out of this relationship and an actual means of escaping it. Heather lived in Manhattan, but she also had a vacation house in the Catskills that was empty for most of the year, and she told me I was welcome to stay there as long as I wanted. In a rare moment of lucidity, I accepted her offer. I was writing copy for a website at the time, and my boss was willing to let me telecommute. Within a few days of Heather's invitation, I had packed my boxes and prepared to move.

The night before I left, Luke and I went out to dinner. We ended up back at his place. We were lying on his bed and I was reading aloud from the Bible—during dinner, I had tried to explain why Mark is my favorite gospel—when he leaned over and kissed me. It turned out that neither of us had a condom, and Luke asked, in a rough whisper, if it would be all right to proceed without. My period had just ended the day before, so I calculated that it would.

This was precisely the third instance of unprotected intercourse I have had in my life. This was also, of course, when I got pregnant.

5.

I found out I was pregnant in early March, but Luke was planning to visit me in the spring, so I decided to wait out the winter before I broke the news to him. I can honestly say that I didn't expect Luke to fall in love with me because I was having his baby. I cannot say that this was not a deeply gratifying vision—one which I entertained with some frequency while I waited to see him—but I imagined other possibilities, too. If the image of familial bliss was my rosiest vision, the darkest was my favorite revenge fantasy, in which Luke, having rejected me and the baby upon learning that I was pregnant, bumps into us many months later, at which point he is overwhelmed by paternal longing when he sees my beautiful, brilliant child. I pretend that I don't even know him and walk on by—a secure, righteously satisfied, and very hip single mother.

The most realistic scenario, I figured, was that, after an initial freak-out, Luke would choose to be our child's father, and that the two of us would figure out how to be parents together. This was more or less what I was anticipating, and I was (more or less) all right with it. My biggest concern was that I would not stop being in love with Luke (the image of his inevitable new girlfriend being involved in my baby's life filled me with particular consternation). I did not imagine that raising a child with Luke would be at all easy, but I had faith in us as parents. I believed we could work through our own problems for our child's sake. I was definitely nervous but I was sustained by a cautious, modest, resilient hope.

Luke and I spent a few pleasant days together. Heather, my hostess, was out of the country, so we stayed at her place in the city. We walked through Central Park, where the trees were just touched with tiny, tender, pale leaves. We went to museums. We ate Indian food. After some initial awkward business about sleeping arrangements—trying to be fair, I offered him the couch—we ended up sleeping together. He didn't produce any condoms, nor did he inquire when I didn't insist upon them, which surprised me, as I had kind of expected that to be the catalyst for my revelation. It wasn't until the night of his departure that I roused the courage to tell him I was pregnant. We were in bed at the time. Luke didn't take the news very well.

6.

I, on the other hand, was preternaturally composed. I knew what I was going to do—I was going to have a baby—and I had prepared myself for an uneasy reaction from Luke. He thrashed about a bit, emotionally and physically, but ultimately he calmed down. After a while, it was possible for us to talk.

He accepted that I wanted to have the baby, but he also asked me to consider having an abortion. He felt trapped, cornered, as if he had been robbed of the choice to be a father. He was only a couple years younger than me, but in some ways he was a lot younger than me. Adulthood, I think, still felt new to him. I assured him that I understood his feelings and that I would consider his request. I did understand how he felt, but I also knew that I was lying when I said I would think about having an abortion. I wanted to get us past his fear and uncertainty, to help him arrive where I already was. I was offering him a gift—a child! I was waiting for him to realize that, like me, he had been blessed.

7.

The night wore on. We talked some more. We both remembered why we liked each other in the first place, and we tried to be kind. Luke acknowledged the reality of the child I was carrying and her place in his life. I acknowledged his fears and found myself capable of patience.

We fell asleep. When we woke up, we went out for breakfast, and then we walked to Penn Station. I cried as Luke got on his train, but he assured me that everything would be all right, and we said good-bye.

I went back to the house in the mountains. The snow was gone by the time I returned, and it was warm enough to open the windows in the daytime. I was so relieved, so hopeful, and the weather seemed to reflect my mood.

I had told a couple of friends as soon as I found out I was pregnant, but I was waiting until after I told Luke, and until I knew whether or not he was going to stick around, before I told anyone else. My friends were excited, my family elated. Luke told his family, too. He had expected them to be angry and disappointed, but if they had any negative feelings, they kept quiet about them. He was surprised and touched by their support.

For the next couple of weeks, Luke and I talked every day. We weren't making any concrete plans yet—we were moving slowly, being careful—but it was good to be able to tell him about my pregnancy, about the morning sickness and the pleasant sleepiness and my total sense of contentment. Everything really was going to be all right. I felt so lucky and so glad.

Then I started bleeding.

8.

It was about ten in the morning when I called my midwife in the city. She didn't seem especially alarmed, but she said she would arrange for some tests for me if I was worried. I asked her to please make the arrangements.

The drive from the mountains to the city took a few hours. I talked to my baby the whole way. I told her that I would take care of her. I told her that we would be all right. I really tried to believe that we would be all right. It was mid-afternoon when I got to the hospital. I found the OB-GYN department and checked myself in. Then, I waited.

I waited forever. When I arrived, there had been a few couples in the waiting room, sitting on hard chairs and holding hands. By six o'clock, I was the only person there. The waiting room was around the corner and down the hall from the reception area, so I went to the reception desk to make sure I hadn't been forgotten; the desk was unattended, and the lights had been turned out. I looked down the corridor, toward the exam rooms, and I didn't see anyone. I tried very hard not to panic. A little bleeding was perfectly normal. Everything was going to be just fine.

I walked down the hallway. I found a woman in scrubs. I explained my situation to her, and asked whether I was ever going to see a doctor. She suggested that I go back to the waiting room.

About half an hour later, another woman in scrubs came for me. She took me to a room lit only by the faint glow of computer monitors. She told me to undress, put on a gown, and sit in a chair with stirrups. Then she left. I did as she told me, and I waited some more.

When she came back, she explained that she was going to put an ultrasound wand inside me. Over her shoulder, I could see a black-and-white image of a bundle of cells. I thought I saw a big head and a tiny curled body and I smiled. This was the first time I had seen my baby. Then the technician typed out a few words on a keyboard, and I could see those, too, as they appeared on the screen. The words were "no fetal heart." She didn't quite look at me when she told me to wait for the doctor.

9.

I could not believe—would not believe—that the words I was reading meant what they obviously did. As I waited for the doctor, I struggled to figure out how they could possibly mean something else. I strained to find some other explanation, but I couldn't.

When the doctor finally arrived, his first words were "I'm sorry." That's when I started crying—howling and keening— and I never heard what came after. All of the sudden, there were several people in the room, and they all seemed to think I was overreacting. A nurse asked me to lift my tongue so that she could give me a little herbal remedy to calm me down. I told her to fuck off. I told them all to fuck off, to leave me alone. My baby was dead. How was I overreacting? I got dressed, still crying and cursing, and I went to the hospital lobby.

First, I called my friend Griffin. He lives in Manhattan,

and I asked him to come to the hospital. He happened to be with Heather at the time. They both came for me and took me back to Griffin's place. Then I called Luke. I told him that I had lost the baby, and that I wanted to go home, that I wanted to be with my mom and my dad and my sister in Ohio, and that I didn't think I could drive myself. He left work early, and started the long drive from Michigan to New York. He got to Griffin's apartment in the East Village in the early hours of the morning. He slept for a while. We went out for breakfast. And then we set out for Ohio.

10.

Women who have had babies say that, yes, the pain is terrible, but you forget it as soon as you hold your baby in your arms.

Having never had a baby, I don't know about that. I can't compare the pain of a miscarriage to the pain of childbirth, but I can say that the pain I experienced was not what my doctor told me to expect. He had said it would be like a bad case of cramps, like intense menstrual discomfort. It was not like that at all. It was much worse, and each time the pain came, I felt the urge to push, and this travesty of labor was worse than any physical hurt.

The doctor had also told me that when I finally expelled the contents of my uterus I wouldn't recognize anything resembling a baby. He wasn't quite right about that, either. I had been studying prenatal development since I first knew I was pregnant, imagining my own child's transformations as the weeks passed. I recognized the gestational sac when I saw it—after I felt the last, fierce, clenching wave of pain, after I gave a final, terrible push.

I held it in the palm of my hand. It was small and round and dark, like a plum. That was the last I saw of my baby.

11.

For a long time after my miscarriage, I couldn't experience her as anything but an absence. I hadn't just lost a baby. I also lost everything I had discovered when I still had her: the joy, the wonder, the knowledge of the absolute and astonishing goodness of being alive. I lost motherhood, too, and the awesome sense of certainty it gave me. I lost a future that I had wanted more than I've ever wanted anything.

12.

I moved back to Ann Arbor, and Luke was very helpful to me in the weeks immediately after the miscarriage. He drove me to doctor's appointments, held my hand while I cried, and listened when I talked about the baby. He had a new girlfriend, though, and she did not much like the idea of me, so it wasn't long before he was out of my life. At first this abandonment made me angry and sad, and the knowledge that Luke was with someone else wasn't easy to take. Looking back, though, I can appreciate how hard this time must have been for Luke, how conflicted he must have been, and I am thankful that he was by my side when I needed him most. I can appreciate that, having decided to be my baby's father, he fulfilled his responsibility as best he could even when the baby was gone.

In fact, my anger and disappointment didn't last that long after Luke disappeared. I soon stopped caring about anyone or anything, and that included him. I retreated from life for a long time after my miscarriage. I took a leave of absence from my job. Grieving became my only occupation. I stopped talking to friends and family. I isolated myself, but, even when I was around other people, I felt disconnected.

13.

When what would have been the baby's due date drew near, I called Luke and asked him if he would spend the day with me, and he agreed. I told him what I'd been going through since the miscarriage, and for the first time I asked him whether he had experienced the miscarriage as a loss. He said he had; he had started to create his own vision of the future before it happened, one that involved philosophical discussions with a precociously curious child and violin lessons. It helped me to know this. It helped me to know that my baby was a person to someone besides me.

14.

It's possible that, if not for the pregnancy and the miscarriage, I would have been able to regard my relationship with Luke as just another romantic misadventure—slightly torturous, yes, and rather embarrassing in retrospect, but not that different from various other amorous blunders I've survived. The baby made things more complicated, and certainly more intense. Now, it seems to me that, for a long time after my miscarriage, giving up on Luke felt like giving up on the baby. He was my only living connection to her, and I didn't want to lose that, too.

I did get over him, though, and, when I did, I decided it was time to start dating again. I answered a few personal ads posted on TheOnion.com and Salon.com. I flirted via e-mail with a few men who looked promising. I set up a few dates.

On my first date with Ted—a college professor, a political scientist with a bone-dry sense of humor and a truly impressive record collection—he took me to see a couple of bands I'd never heard of, and I loved them both. Afterward, I canceled the dates I had planned with other men. That was four years ago, and we've been together ever since.

Everything that was hard with Luke is easy with Ted. We challenge each other, but we also support each other. We have an emotional accord that Luke and I never shared, a kind of love I've never known with anyone else: passionate, but also comfortable, secure, and sustainable. These words may sound boring unless one has experienced both their absence and their presence. It doesn't take a whole lot of effort or drama for us to be happy together. I can hardly believe my good luck.

We got married in Ann Arbor, at the county courthouse, almost two years ago. Ted knew about my pregnancy, my miscarriage, and my definite desire for children before he proposed. At first he was dubious about fatherhood—it was the only serious issue between us and marriage—but when he found himself having an imaginary argument with our hypothetical teenaged offspring, he realized that, without even knowing it, he had decided he could do it. Our baby, a girl, is due in a couple of months.

15.

It would be nice for this story, the story of my miscarriage, to have a happy ending. It would be nice if this new baby made up for that lost baby, if my current happiness erased my prior grief. But that's not exactly how it is. It's true that I stopped grieving for my first baby a long time ago, but I'll never forget that baby—the joy of discovering her, the anguish of losing her, and the slow process of learning to live without her.

This pregnancy is not like the first. My elation has been colored—not diminished, but informed—by my experience of loss. I am a little wiser this time, a little more cautious in my joy. I am hopeful, and I am excited. I am aware of the fragility of this miracle I'm carrying, and I am so grateful to have another chance.

The Missing

Rachel Hall

The first miscarriage was a mistake. Or, rather, the pregnancy was a mistake. We hadn't planned it. "A happy accident," my husband and I said when we announced the pregnancy to our parents. I won't lie; there was ambivalence, too. Is any second child not anticipated with some ambivalence? Those sleepless nights of early infanthood, the exhausting vigilance, the high-stakes guesswork—they get burned into the brain, turned into something solid to stumble over. This, at least, is the way it happened for me. I had thought I was done after one child. I was thirty-eight years old. My daughter was nearly six, she could tie her shoes, play happily by herself, wipe her own bottom. My brain and body felt like they were mostly my own again.

But there was joy, too, when I confirmed that I was pregnant on that cold January day—the house quiet, my daughter at school, my husband at work. Waiting for the pink line on the pregnancy test to appear, I knew I'd be disappointed if it didn't. And then, there it was, clear and bright. I was pregnant. A mistake, but as my mother-in-law says of her fourth child, my husband, "the best mistake I ever made."

Naturally I cleaned up my act at this point: no more coffee, no more wine with dinner, no beer with friends after a movie (there were no movies, actually, since I was too tired to go out). No more serotonin reuptake inhibitors. (Goodbye, happiness!) No more coloring my hair. I monitored my diet with vigilance. My mind carefully calculated calories, protein, vitamins, but it also leapt ahead—by weeks and months—until I was holding my baby, nursing her in the quiet nursery I would make for her in the sunny room off our bedroom. I bought things, too: a pair of butter-yellow fleece booties, two cotton sleepers, and a maternity blouse (I wasn't going to frump my way through this pregnancy as I had my last one).

At my ultrasound appointment, scheduled for dating purposes, I lay on the paper-draped table in the dark examination room, the condomed strobe searching inside me. I was about eleven weeks pregnant according to the date of my last period, but we needed a more exact date for the complicated genetics tests I'd signed on for. I watched the glowing computer screen, but I didn't really know what I was looking for. It had been six years, after all, since my last ultrasound—and then, I'd only had one. Even the certified technician, presumably with years of experience under her belt, had to call in a doctor to tell me there was no heartbeat. My baby wasn't a baby.

How could this be? In my heart, I knew the baby to be a girl, to be named Ruby, a sister for Maude. There was a terrible gap between what I'd imagined and what was happening, and as I stood at the edge looking down, it seemed impossible to find my way across. It also felt unfair, *a miscarriage of justice. Our plans miscarried.*

The baby things I bought were easy to return, and I did, or else I gave them away, all except for those soft booties that, even now, when I think of them, can make me cry. But what does it mean to long for something I hadn't even thought I'd wanted, wasn't sure I could handle? Was I perhaps mourning something else? Wishing that I were a better, less ambivalent person, warm and generous, open-armed and eager to meet the needs of many children?

There are no hard and fast rules about when to announce a pregnancy to your five-year-old daughter who has been asking for a sibling. And even if there were rules, we probably wouldn't have followed them. My husband and I were confident, brazen even, I see now. We hadn't even tried to get pregnant, and look at us! We told our parents immediately, then friends. At first we didn't tell Maude, but one day, when I was about six weeks pregnant, she asked again for a baby sister and I couldn't hold back any longer. "You're going to be a big sister," I told her, and my mind did it again—leapt forward, imagined Maude as my little helper, fetching bottles, singing for the baby in her sweet, clear voice. I saw Maude on the couch holding the swaddled baby while I gazed down at them, my children. I savored that phrase: *my children.*

"Mommy," Maude said one morning in early March as we

waited for her school bus to arrive, "you're going to have to get some of those big lady clothes, you know."

My breath made a cloud as I laughed. "Maternity clothes, yes," I said. "A good idea."

"And Mommy," she said, "Maybe we can both be this baby's mother."

She talked about the baby a lot during the month that followed, how she would teach her things, show her things. She drew pictures for the baby. It was a time of luscious anticipation. When I worried about how we'd manage with two children, I'd think of Maude's excitement. I was giving her a sibling, which she very much wanted. Surely that was worth more than anything. She'd have someone with whom to complain about me and her father, to describe in detail our annoying tics and bad habits, our disastrous taste in furnishings or movies or vacation spots.

Still, I worried. For two years after Maude's birth, I'd hardly written a word. I'd been too tired, too preoccupied, too anxious about my new duties and responsibilities. I steeped myself in childcare literature, and not surprisingly the tone and language of the experts inspired more anxiety and no short stories. Now those lost writing years weighed on me: I had a novel to finish, a collection of stories to revise, all kinds of projects for which I'd need my wits and plenty of rest.

Another reason I hadn't wanted a second child was my own experience as the eldest of two children. While growing up, my brother and I had plenty of books and toys, lessons and camps, family vacations to the see Fort Ticonderoga or the home of Laura Ingalls Wilder. However, my parents were constantly distracted by their troubled marriage, and my brother and I battled each other for their attention. When we fought, we were told to work it out on our own. Good advice, I suppose, if one is given a model of such behavior. In my mind, having only one child had seemed like a way to prevent this paucity of love. But here was Maude showing me what love could do. It didn't have to be stretched tight and thin; it could expand exponentially, wildly combining and recombining.

There are few things harder than telling a child about death. Technically I know this isn't a death. There is nothing even vaguely resembling a baby in the bloody mess that gets flushed down the toilet, but there is no other way to frame this discussion. There are no better words. How could I answer Maude's questions when I had so many myself? Why had this happened? Was it something I'd done wrong? A *misdeed*? I don't remember how we told her, only that we cried together. And that later, she suggested we "try and try again" to make a baby, our words of encouragement when she makes a mistake reading or drawing or building.

We did try again, as Maude suggested. We planned another pregnancy, but fearfully, the anticipation reined in, quiet surrounding it. I bought nothing, told few people, as if this could prevent the unspeakable, make it hurt less should anything go wrong. Even Maude was kept in the dark this time. I had held on to all our baby equipment, because to get rid of it seemed too final, and now I was glad I did. In the attic we had a crib and bassinet, a changing table, and carefully labeled boxes of baby clothes. The basement was stocked with a Jolly Jumper, a swing, board books, outgrown toys, and a brand-new stroller that looked like an old-fashioned pram. I could imagine pushing that stroller, my newborn inside, milky and sated, as I step into dappled sunlight.

　　　　　　　　　　　⟨ ⟩

When I miscarried for the second time, it was easy to say "That's it—I'm done with this racket." Enough is enough. But lately, I've begun thinking that we could try again. Maybe three is the charm. According to my midwife, my chances of another miscarriage have increased only about 5 percent. She also tells me I shouldn't wait much longer if I'm going to try to conceive again. My eggs are old. In her voice, I hear caution and resignation. She doesn't want me to get my hopes up.

I don't completely trust my impulse to try again, though. Are my fantasies about another child really mine? Or is it someone else's dream, a prescription for the American family and my womanly role within it? Maybe I'm trying to pin a happy ending on this story, but surely there are happy endings besides the one that would have a new baby nuzzling at my breast. And I understand that there is no guarantee of staving off loneliness for my daughter, not with one sibling or ten. Perhaps it is just this: Having begun this project, a well-trained part of me demands follow-through. *If at first you don't succeed . . .*

　　　　　　　　　　　⟨ ⟩

One Saturday my small family and I decide to see a matinee. The movie is a comedy, a remake of a 1950s favorite, complete with tons of children, traditional gender roles, and a kind of slapstick which makes me tired. Leaving the theater after the film, I asked Maude what she thought about all those kids in one family. "Too much noise," she said, "and mess."

"Wouldn't it be fun, though?" I asked.

"Maybe," she said.

Just as I was when I was her age, Maude is certain that she will be a mother one day. "How many children do you think you'd like to have?" I ask now, taking the hand of my one and only. It is warm and small in my own.

"I don't know," she says, furrowing her brow. "Maybe three, or two, or one."

Getting into the car, we agree that she has plenty of time to decide.

Piece of Cake

Rachel Zucker

"I feel really, *really* sick," I told the nurse practitioner when the day of my first OB visit finally arrived.

"Are you keeping food down?" she asked, wrapping the blood pressure cuff tightly around my upper arm.

"I'm not actually throwing up, just gagging and retching. On the subway, in elevators, I feel sick every minute of the night and day. I can barely—"

"Wait," she said, holding up a finger, listening through her stethoscope. "Perfect!" she said, recording my blood pressure. She noted everything in the chart, including the fact that I was ten pounds over my pre-pregnancy weight.

"Morning sickness is a good sign. Really. Your body's hard at work making hormones." She smiled. She suggested I drink ginger ale.

Ginger ale? I'd already tried ginger ale. I'd also tried saltines, raw almonds, Sea-Bands, ginger tea, ginger candy, mint tea, mint candy, meditation, waking up in the middle of the night to eat so that my blood sugar level didn't go down, eating before I got out of bed, eating small frequent protein snacks throughout the day, cutting out greasy foods, cutting out sugar.

"I sleep with a glass of ginger ale, a packet of saltines, a jar of peanut butter, and a puke bucket next to my bed," I told her.

The nurse smiled again and called in the obstetrician.

"Piece of cake," said the OB, looking over the chart, "Piece . . . of . . . cake. . . ." She smiled as she made notes. Most of my OB's clients were professional Manhattanite women in their late thirties or forties. In the waiting room, sitting next to all of them, I had felt like a pregnant teenager, even though I was twenty-six years old. My husband, twenty-five, looked even more out of place among the expectant fathers, many of whom were old enough to be *his* father.

The OB smiled at me; she smiled at my husband. I had looked forward to this visit, hoping to find sympathy and perhaps a solution for the unremitting nausea I'd experienced over the past six weeks. I was sick of feeling so sick and wanted the doctor to know that. The nurse just kept smiling at me.

The nurse wheeled over a contraption with a monitor and dials and a white plastic phallus-shaped stick. She covered the white plastic wand, as she called it, with a latex shield that looked like a loose condom and lavishly squirted the shield with thick clear gel.

"It won't hurt the—?" I was embarrassed to even ask such a question. Obviously these smiling women were not in the business of harming pregnant women or fetuses. Still, it seemed so invasive, the long white wand.

The OB looked at me and smiled a patient, condescending

smile. "Your uterus is like this," she made a tight fist, "closed. Get it?" She explained that even though I said I was sure I knew when I'd conceived (she obviously didn't believe me) it was important to accurately date my pregnancy. "You know how sonar works?" she asked, but by then she wasn't really talking to me. She was checking the connections and fiddling with the dials. "Good, good . . . good . . . hmmm. . . ."

I wondered if "hmmm" was different from "good"?

"Well . . . hmmm . . . ," she said again, and adjusted the controls. She moved the wand inside me.

"This," she said, pointing to a black ovoid shape on the screen, "this, here, is a gestational sac. That's all you can really see at this stage. From the size of the sac I would say that you are indeed about eight weeks pregnant." I felt vindicated, proud. "And this," she moved the wand slightly and a black shape slid away and then appeared again, "is another sac. Let's see if I can get them both on the screen at once."

"Them?" said my husband.

"You, daddy, may be having twins."

"Whoa," said my husband.

Huh, I thought.

"No wonder you feel so sick," she said to me, "twice the hormones."

She pointed at the two sacs, which bloomed in and out of focus on the screen like craters on a moonscape. I nodded to indicate that I understood what she was saying, although I was barely listening. Twins. *Huh.*

The next appointment, three weeks later, confirmed the presence of twins. The doctor heard two healthy heartbeats on the Doppler, saw two well-formed sacs, two blinking fetuses. Though I wasn't quite at the end of my first trimester, the chances for miscarriage had dropped dramatically and the OB gave us the go-ahead to tell our friends and families.

My husband announced the news to my father over dinner with a proud, devious smile. Soon afterward, he told everyone else we knew, as well as many people we didn't know. My husband seemed to enjoy the response he got—the surprise, the worry, the wide-eyed stares. Everyone was fascinated by the idea of twins. My husband knew, of course, that having twins was a function of either my ovaries having released two eggs in the case of fraternal twins or of the egg splitting after fertilization in the case of identical (both circumstances caused by my body and not by his), but he touted the news as if the presence of twins reflected his powerful virility. He made sure that people knew that we'd gotten pregnant in our second month of trying, that we hadn't used fertility drugs, that his mother had twin brothers.

I let him brag. I was scared as hell.

For as long as I can remember, I've suffered intense bouts of baby lust. A pregnant woman passing by on the street was enough to make me lose my train of thought. I stared at women's bellies the way some people stare at models' bodies: I wanted what they had, and I wanted it badly. During the first few years of my relationship with my husband (then my boyfriend) I'd managed to keep my baby lust in check, although I often whispered "look at her!" when I saw a pregnant woman. But the desire to have a child became more intense every year. After we had been living together for a few years I told him I was ready to have a baby, and I didn't care about getting married. He was adamant that we not have a baby without being married, though, so six months later I proposed to him, and he accepted.

My husband provided the sperm necessary to spark our blastula into being, but I have to admit that I was the motivating force in our baby-making. I was a bulldozer on the road to parenthood, clearing the path of all perceived obstacles including his doubts about whether he was ready to be a father. I'm not saying that I lied, at least not consciously, but the picture of parenthood that I painted for my husband, prepregnancy, was like a Monet painting of a garden—all light and color and mood, without the specific details of weeds, blossoms, or brambles.

"We'll still travel and go out to eat," I promised, "not like all those silly parents with their uptight schedules. Our baby will be good in restaurants because we'll go out so often that he or she will be used to such things. You know, a baby really doesn't take up any space at all, doesn't even eat food for the first year, really. . . ." I believed most of this myself. I'd babysat from the time I was ten. I'd been a mother's helper, a day camp counselor, a preschool teacher's assistant. In college I'd majored in child development, earning course credits for interning at several daycare centers. Being good with kids was something I valued highly about myself.

Although I knew that being a mom wasn't always easy, I couldn't imagine why it would be hard. Not for someone like me—I was an expert.

This was back in the days when I expected that pregnancy would be an ideal time to start new hobbies, like learning to cook authentic Chinese food or knit elaborate sweaters. I pictured myself parading around in flimsy white nightgowns or bathing suits with horizontal stripes. I thought pregnancy would be a blissfully contemplative time, a time that would enable me—a college-level teacher/writer who believed that each minute not spent teaching should be spent writing—to relax, because I would feel, for the first time in my life, that every waking and sleeping moment was so wonderfully productive, important, and pregnant (excuse the pun) with meaning that I'd already accomplished something merely by breathing, eating, and thinking positive thoughts.

⁓

As I passed the end of the first trimester, however, I was still unremittingly ill. I was practically an invalid. I couldn't drive; I couldn't go downstairs to get the mail without retching in the elevator. I was barely managing my teaching job. And contemplation? Forget it. Between the bone-aching exhaustion and the suspicion that my brain had been replaced by Mallomars (my OB called this "placenta head"), I felt about as contemplative and accomplished as a cotton ball.

But even worse than the physical and cognitive changes, or the dashed fantasy of pregnancy-as-bliss, was the terror about birth and motherhood that had begun to grip me. I had felt so confident about having a baby. I had made a hard sell to my husband and was ready to stand by my promises. But all that was before I found out that I was pregnant with twins.

In books about multiple pregnancies, women, naked and hugely pregnant with "multiples," posed proudly. To me they appeared impossibly, unnaturally proportioned. One was standing on a scale that read "190" despite her obviously thin frame. She looked as if she'd swallowed a large suitcase. These women seemed to be on the verge of bursting at the seams, splitting down the *linea negra* that ran from their belly buttons to their pelvises. I couldn't bear to look at the picture of the woman thirty-eight weeks pregnant with triplets.

The photos of women nursing twins also unnerved me. The books strongly recommended tandem nursing (nursing two babies at once) saying that in the first few weeks, a mother of multiples might otherwise spend almost all day and night nursing. They advised keeping a notebook to record how long each baby nursed, as it would be impossible to keep track otherwise. There were illustrations of helpful nursing pillows and photographs of women nursing twins using a "double clutch," a "double football," or a more traditional "crisscross" nursing hold. I was ashamed of how the pictures made me feel: uneasy, nervous, vaguely disgusted. The mothers' breasts were enormous, as big as cantaloupes, and I could not look at them clutching their babies' tiny heads without thinking that they looked like mother animals nursing a litter. The thought of nursing one baby felt lovely, beautiful, doable to me, but the idea of nursing two, particularly at the same time, made me feel anxious, tired, and exploited.

It wasn't just the nursing. It was everything. One baby seemed to take up no space at all, but when I imagined two, I pictured me and my husband huddled together in the only corner of our apartment not piled high with strollers and highchairs and cribs and baby swings, like refugees from our former life.

⁓

At fifteen weeks we went back to the OB. No bleeding, no cramping, still nauseous as ever. The doctor was quite pleased with my progress, although she chastised me for putting on so much weight. "Let's just check," she said and wheeled over the sonogram machine. Quickly one fetus appeared on the screen. The fetus was much more developed than it had been in the last sonogram. I was thrilled to be able to see the head, arms, legs, and bumpy spinal column quite clearly. The fetus fluttered and rolled. "Hold still, little baby," the OB said, "I need to measure you." She placed the star-shaped cursor on the screen over the baby's head and dragged it down to the baby's butt, making a dotted line appear on the screen. "Got it," she said. She pressed a button and a printout slid out of the machine. She handed it to my husband. She slid the transducer to one side. Shadowy shapes appeared and disappeared and then suddenly I saw it: the other fetus.

I knew right away that something was wrong. The fetus's head was turned away from the transducer. It was still. Perfectly still. "Hmmm," the OB said.

"What is it? What's wrong with—? Why isn't it—?" I said.

"Let's just see here," said the OB. She moved the transducer, trying to get a different view. She used her fingers to prod, strongly, at the fetus through my abdomen.

The fetus didn't move.

"Maybe he . . . or she, it, whatever is . . . sleeping?" said my husband. The doctor and I ignored him. She swiveled the screen away from me so that I couldn't see it. She adjusted the dials on the machine, slid the transducer over my stomach, prodded and poked, pushed and pressed on my full bladder.

"I'm going to need to send you to a sonogram center. I think that one fetus has stopped out. I'd like you to go tonight." Her voice was even and emotionless. Stopped out? I was crying. My husband awkwardly touched my shoulder.

"We were only trying for one," he said.

⁓

The technician wouldn't let my husband come with me into the examining room. He wouldn't let me look at the screen. He wouldn't answer my questions. He offered me tissues to wipe my face and blow my nose. After what seemed like a long time, he called in the doctor. "See here? And here? This?" the technician said to the doctor, pointing at the screen. The doctor nodded. The technician handed me a wad of paper towels, pointed at my white-whale stomach, which was covered in gel and said, "Why don't you get cleaned up?"

My husband was ushered into the room. The blue paper gown, wet from tears and snot and gel, barely covered me. "Is it dead?" my husband asked, pointing at my stomach.

I loved him for asking, for saying the word "dead" out loud. Although tears ran down my cheeks, I felt, in the eerie fluorescent light of the examining room, numb, silenced, dissociated. My husband's bumbling naïveté, his innocent way of talking too much and asking obvious questions, was the only weapon we had to pierce through the stultifying and isolating medical façade.

"You can't say dead exactly," said the doctor, shifting from one foot to the other, "Is your liver alive? Your kidney?"

I didn't want to talk about it, so I sat in the rocking chair in our darkened bedroom and through the half-closed door listened to my husband repeat the story over and over to our parents and stepparents, grandparents and friends.

"It turns out it's quite common," he said. "It's called 'vanishing twin syndrome' . . . the OB says that the fetal tissue will be reabsorbed into her body . . . yeah I know, kind of creepy . . . no, no, the other fetus, uh, baby should be fine . . . no nothing, she felt nothing . . . no, no bleeding . . . yeah, happens a lot, I guess—something like one out of eight pregnancies start out as twins, with these early sonograms now . . . yeah, they said probably stopped developing, about a week or two ago . . . yeah, okay, or, well, not so good really, no, she doesn't want to talk right now . . . yeah, I'll tell her, we know, we know, we love you, too." After a while he started to sound almost upbeat. He was getting the hang of saying "fetal tissue" and "vanishing twin syndrome." It was becoming a story, a routine. I heard him say, "Yeah, well, there's some relief in it, too."

A few weeks passed. My teaching semester ended. It was December break. The OB insisted that we not go, as we had planned, with my father and stepmother to Umbria, Italy. I was surprised. "Air travel is extremely dehydrating," she explained to us, "and I really would not recommend a trip right now." When I asked her whether I should be worried about the pregnancy, she was adamant that everything was fine, that everything would be fine. "Stop worrying so much," she said to me, "you'll make yourself crazy. This happens all the time." On the other hand, she advised me not to do exercise more strenuous than a brisk walk. Again, I was surprised; she had often bragged to us about her many patients who ran or played tennis through their seventh month. I asked her whether a multiple pregnancy was more or less high-risk than a vanishing twin pregnancy. "Look," she said, "I've done enough hand-holding for one day. You're going to have to trust me. Everything is fine." Clearly, my pregnancy was no longer a piece of cake.

I spent most of December lying in bed or on the couch. I watched television, tried to read, wondered whether I should change obstetricians. (Of course I should have switched from the moment she first dismissed my fears and concerns, but I was young and naïve and my husband liked her.) I became obsessed by a news story about a man in the Balkans who had been buried alive in a mass grave. A few weeks later my great-aunt was diagnosed with pancreatic cancer and given three months to live. The same day, during an appointment, the

OB mentioned that if I were to "expel" the stopped-out fetus it might be dangerous to the "happy twin." I lay in bed trying to keep the "fetal material" inside me though I had no idea how to do that. I thought about my great-aunt's cancer growing inside her, the thing they could not take out. I thought about the dissolving fetal tissue inside me being reabsorbed by my body, by the living fetus, and tried to keep everything—life, death—inside me.

I was haunted by the fact that I had felt nothing, nothing at all when the fetus died inside me. What if something was wrong with the other fetus, the "happy twin" as the OB continued to call my developing baby? How would I know? My body was unreliable. I couldn't protect my baby; I was already a bad mother. I lay on the couch and watched television. I lay on the couch and tried not to think, "I have a dead baby inside me."

The phone rang with people speaking in euphemisms and offering up clichés such as "these things happen for a reason." I knew the well-wishers meant to say that the fetus had died because of a chromosomal abnormality or a congenital defect. It couldn't, shouldn't have been born, they were trying, politely, to say. And though I believed this, the phrase got on my nerves. I had to stop myself from responding with hostile comebacks such as "Well, maybe the *reason* this happened is that I didn't *want* the baby to live because twins are more than I could handle." Or "Perhaps when the baby heard all the people around me using stupid, trite clichés like *things happen for a reason* the baby thought life wasn't worth living."

As a joke my husband and I started using the phrase at inappropriate times. If my husband said he couldn't find the Scotch tape, I would say, with a look of grave concern, my voice dripping with false sympathy, "These things happen for a reason." After a while the refrain "these things happen for a reason" led to a free-for-all of miscarriage-related clichés. I'd come home to find a note from my husband by the phone: "Tom called to say he's sorry about the baby and suggests we remember that a stitch in time does indeed save nine." Late at night I'd whisper to my husband, "You know, I was feeling really freaked out about what's going on but then I called Joan and she said, 'Don't put off until tomorrow what you can do today,' and I felt much better."

At eighteen weeks and four days I started to feel the baby move. At first, light and fluttery, like a bubble in seltzer, then, after a few more weeks, I could discern distinct movements: rolling, kicking, stretching. He (we had by then found out the baby was a boy) felt active but calm. I can't quite explain it, but even when he kicked me hard in the ribs he seemed peaceful. A shadow of anxiety still clung to the pregnancy, but the sixteen-week sonogram had revealed no abnormalities, and feeling the baby move was tremendously reassuring. If he was moving, he was alive.

It was awkward when I ran into people who thought I was still having twins. Most made a quick apology—"Oh, I didn't know . . ."—and changed the subject. One woman said, "Are you sure? You're so big!" But, for the most part, my OB's promise that things would be fine seemed to be coming true. Three weeks before my estimated due date the doctor suggested we induce labor. She was concerned that the placenta, as a "twins' placenta," might not be functioning well. The baby seemed to be slowing down a little, I was already partially effaced and dilated and, perhaps not insignificantly, the OB's daughter was graduating from Harvard Law School the following week. After two days of failing to start labor by drinking castor oil, going on long walks, or employing my husband's conjugal services, I agreed to the induction.

~

This is not a story that ends with a moving description of what I did with the cute pair of twin's overalls we had received early on as a gift, because I can't remember what I did with them. After my son was born I was subsumed in the experience of mothering him: the details, the emotions, the banalities, the extraordinariness of it all. I stopped staring at the walls and listening to my heartbeat and started watching my child sleep, listening to him breathe. My son eclipsed almost all traces of the outside world.

At night, though, I still dreamed about my son's "lost" twin. In one variation of the recurring dreams I have, I take my son to visit his grandmother. When I arrive at my mother's brownstone apartment I find the *other* baby. Another baby? I'm confused. All this time I left this second baby with my mother? How could I have done such a thing? I realize, to my horror, that I'd forgotten about this baby and now there he is: big, pale, angry, abandoned. In all my dreams the "lost" child is male, highly verbal, bigger than my tiny son. He is always angry. I am always ashamed.

~~~

Some doctors estimate that between 30 and 80 percent of all people were once twins. Another estimate is that one in eight pregnancies begins as a multiple pregnancy. Before the advent of early sonography these twins went unnoticed by midwives and obstetricians. The fact that I briefly thought I was going to have twins is a fluke of technology, and mainstream modern medicine would have me believe that the whole thing is no big deal.

My dreams, my poems, and my heart believe otherwise. The knowledge, the language, and the image of my lost fetus colored my experience of pregnancy and childbirth and perhaps even my perceptions of my son. The lost twin made me see my living fetus as "surviving" rather than simply developing. I thought of him as imperiled, fragile, besieged, possibly traumatized.

I was relieved to have one child instead of twins, but I wouldn't have called what I felt when I saw the ultrasound image of my dead child "relief." When I saw the human-shaped form inside me, its spinal cord like a loosely strung strand of pearls, so impossibly, unnaturally still, I felt a thud, a shock. It was a hot, fierce sensation, like the sound of the slap of an oar hitting the dark ocean. The sight of my dead baby knocked the breath out of me and eviscerated my (naïve) confidence.

The OB had looked inside me in order to date my pregnancy, to measure my fetus, to line up the facts and figures. What the picture revealed was, in part, a reminder of how much we do not know. There is something frightening about being pregnant, as well as many things that are beautiful. Science doesn't have the words for it. Medicine doesn't have the language for it. Psychology doesn't have a formula to analyze it. Even poetry and art can't fully describe it. Throughout my pregnancy I was surprised by the inability of medicine, however powerful, to quantify and define the birth process. There are slippery, subtle, and important differences between an embryo, fetus, newborn, or baby, and on the other hand, something that has vanished, disappeared, died, been absorbed, or stopped out. Why is there no single English word to describe the loss of something you didn't think you wanted. Forfeiture? Riddance? Cessation? There is no easy way to describe the imbroglio of emotions that grew up around me during those difficult months. I was angry with the dead baby because he (both his life and death) threatened my living child. Yet I felt ashamed of my anger at this blameless fetus, and horribly guilty for having failed to keep them both alive.

The day after my son was born the OB told me that I had no idea how lucky I was. The pathology on the placenta showed that my twins were "mono-mono" twins, identical twins sharing one sac, a high-risk pregnancy. When I reminded her that initially she had seen two sacs, not one, she brushed the question away. To this day I'm not sure whether I once carried identical twins or fraternal twins, whether the pregnancy was high-risk or a common occurrence. What I do know is that my child, my singleton, is unique in the world just as my experience of becoming a mother was radically personal and specific and amazing. My beautiful, brilliant son is perfect, whole, and more than enough to make us a family. He is also, though I have spent more than five years caring for him and loving him, ultimately as unknowable and strange to me as he was when I first saw his shadowy shape on the monitor. I know, too, that while I will always try to keep him safe I am incapable of protecting him from the all the dangers and grief of the world. Of course, I know how lucky I am.

PART III

Mourning and Moving On

The Scattering

Sylvia Brownrigg

I t was such a small box.

There was never any way that the box would have the magnitude and significance of our loss, but there was nevertheless something awful about how out of scale this small, rectangular, white plastic container was when we were finally given it. "Must have been a small baby," commented the woman at the crematorium, with less tact than I'd hoped for from someone in her position.

The crematorium offices were some distance from us, in an outer county in Northern California, along a dingy, unpromising street. As with so much of our experience with Linnaeus, my husband Sedge and I were accompanied by our son, Samuel, not yet two, and my stepson, Henry, seven. There was a certain need to keep up appearances. Samuel was, as always, cheerful; to this day he does not know that he lost a brother, that he spent hours as a toddler laughing up into my weeping face. Henry, on the other hand, was curious and philosophical.

"I think we should just drive up there now, after we get

them," Henry said. He and his father and I were talking about when to scatter Linnaeus's ashes. We had already decided where we would do this—up at Lake Tahoe, as Sedge and I had walked there together shortly before Linnaeus died. I had had Samuel on my back in a backpack that September afternoon, while my belly moved and bulged with the baby within. The lake, of course, is beautiful, clear and expansive and circled by grand, forgiving mountains. We wanted to take him back there.

"It's too long a drive," I said. We had come from Henry's school, collecting him and driving on to try to find the offices before they closed for the afternoon. I was not yet ready for the scattering. It was only November. Linnaeus had died on the second day of October. I knew there was not going to be anything particularly revelatory about the ashes (although I did not imagine the small white box), but I wanted still to hold on to them, for some weeks at least, some months, before we released them back into the world. Before we found a place to lay what remained of him to rest.

It had taken so long for just this, this meager collection. We had already had salt ground into our wounds by the hospital, its incompetence and carelessness. That evening after Linnaeus had died, the kind nurse allowed us to say good-bye to him and then removed him, this diminutive boy, to whatever fate awaits bodies that have stilled and become lifeless.

I did not allow myself to think about it, actually, what happened to Linnaeus when they took him away. I knew we had signed something (When? Who? Did I sign it, or did Sedge?) saying that we wanted the body cremated, that we would not be burying him. And I knew from attending the support group meetings that any ritual we might have would help us, afterward. That is the sort of thing they tell you at support group meetings. The good folks there (Henry used to call the people at these meetings "the Criers," when I told him what they were like, couples sitting around a table weeping) hand over truths you may not yet have come to: Rituals are important; you should have some kind of service, whatever feels right to you; you'll find that it will help. *I see*, you say to yourself, making a silent note in your numb, bewildered state. Rituals help, do they? I will have to bear that in mind.

So, several weeks after Linnaeus died, moved by another couple's story of a beautiful, simple service they had held for their baby, that had involved the lighting of candles with friends, I called the hospital to find out about collecting the ashes. Hmmm, a woman said to me on the phone. Has the crematorium not been in touch with you directly? No, they hadn't. They should have been. Hmmm. She would have to make inquiries.

That is how we found out, a month or so on from his death, that Linnaeus had been forgotten somewhere in the hospital morgue. Bureaucratic oversight. Institutional error. *We're very sorry, of course*, they had told us.

It was another occasion for grief and rage. We both felt so betrayed, and at the same time so neglectful, as if we had let our child down. Sedge was far more eloquent about it than I. "You have desecrated the memory of our son," he bellowed at a woman from Patient Services. The bellow was inevitable; again, an effort to make the expression somehow proportionate to the strength of feeling. I'd have rent my garments if I could have. "You have failed in the most basic task any of us have, including a hospital: You have failed to honor the dead." Suddenly I had been given a new image to hold on to: our tiny too-soon son cold on a slab in some abandoned drawer in the basement of the hospital. I have no idea how hospitals work. It was not pleasant to imagine. They were very apologetic. We were urged to write letters. A woman from Patient Services sent a note of regret, and some flowers.

So they were ready for us, finally. The crematorium offices. It was a shabby little room up some dark stairs. It felt like we were visiting a second-rate private investigator about some shady affair rather than making a family outing to collect the remains of our son. We got to the small room, whereupon Samuel immediately started to seek objects for play and destruction. Henry was open-faced and even-tempered. The woman had us sign a form. She made it clear that though, strictly speaking, there were places we were not meant to scatter these ashes, once we had signed to acknowledge their receipt it was no longer the crematorium's business what we did with them. She handed over the box. That's when she said, "Must have been a small baby," and what I don't remember well now is whether I held myself together for Henry's sake, or whether, as so often then, I dissolved.

A few mornings later, up early with Henry, Sedge urged Henry to help decorate the box. It was so starkly white. I came down to find the container warmed, humanized, by their colorful drawings and letters. *LBT. Linnaeus Bell Thomson. Samuel Henry Sylvia and Sedge love you and miss you.*

We still have the box. It sits on a shelf near the plates and the cookies, a fine film clinging to its interior, what was left after the scattering.

~

I had not wanted to be pregnant. I had not expected to be pregnant just ten months after the birth of our son. It was carelessness. (Yes, we were guilty of it, too.) In a bemused later moment I blamed our predicament on my friend in New York who was undergoing IVF treatments; after hearing in detail about her uncomfortable ordeal it seemed to me next to impossible that anyone should ever get pregnant, and therefore it was safe for me to count on the fact that I was still nursing, the calendar's certain distance from any fleeting instant of fertility I might have.

I was wrong.

My husband and I greeted the news with dread and dismay. (How could we have allowed that mistake? What would we do now?) I tried to find some shred of pleasure at the prospect of another pregnancy, and if my husband had felt differently I might have located some, but as it was we were thrust into a dark, argumentative stretch, a still-new couple's coping with an unhappy shock.

It was too soon. We had been through so much already. Two years earlier, after months of mysterious uterine pains followed by an early miscarriage, I had spent some time poised on that knife edge of doubt, wondering if I could successfully carry a child to term at all—even as I got to know the existing child brought swiftly into my life, my exuberant young stepson. My pregnancy with Samuel, when it came, was joyful and miserable and worry-laden. I was sick all the time. It was labeled a high-risk pregnancy, due to a uterine anomaly I have. I was subjected throughout to a battery of tests, some reassuring and some less so, until the healthy baby boy was born in late July. It was now late May. Samuel— lively, adorable, blessed Samuel—had not yet taken his first steps. He was ten months old.

The irony was evident to us both, every step of the way: how much we had wanted Samuel, and struggled through our difficulties to arrive at his birth; how much we resisted the fact of this pregnancy now. I immediately began to feel sick again. Samuel was still up several times a night, and to the exhaustion of his first year was added the tiredness of my early pregnancy. We were both fretful about how we could care for this much family this quickly, how we would be able to give Samuel and Henry the attention they needed after a new baby's arrival. I wondered how I would reclaim my sense of myself as a writer with the unceasing demands of two small children. My husband was thrust into his own specific memories of growing up with his brother, just fifteen months his junior, with whom he has had an estranged and sometimes contentious relationship.

There was an early episode of bleeding, which brought to mind my miscarriage of several years earlier, an occasion of great sorrow. This time I embraced my husband one night as I told him about the blood spots, and he asked me what I felt. I answered, "Grief, and relief." But a scan at the doctor's office showed that all was still fine; the bleeding was not meaningful.

Soon after, the prenatal tests, which had caused us much undue anxiety with Samuel, were performed, and they told us that I was carrying a genetically normal boy. I began to take in the fact that, since we were sure this would be our last child, I would never have a daughter. I was about twelve weeks in at this point, and beginning to accept the idea that we were to have two little boys together, two little brothers, close in age. Sedge, even with his continued bewilderment, always asserted, "We will love him when he comes."

We traveled to Europe, Sweden and England, on a so-called honeymoon trip and to celebrate Samuel's first birthday. In England we visited many friends with children, some with a pair of boys, and I canvassed everyone I knew: How is it to have only boys? What will it be like to have two so close in age? I harvested comfort and congratulation like a desperate farmer of a key crop, gathering stories of brothers who were close, of how much easier it would be, really, to have children the same sex, and both in diapers at once, of how Samuel would learn to love his baby sibling. We told Henry, who was excited. Another boy! That had to be good.

I remember walking around Stockholm with my husband, pushing Samuel in his stroller, constantly watching mothers with their children, scanning the sunny city squares for pairs of blond-headed brothers. We came upon streets named for the famous botanist Carl Linnaeus, and my husband mentioned that as a possible middle name for the baby. That was a good sign. If Sedge was thinking of names, it meant he was beginning to open his heart to this new person. For my part, though I was wearied now by the combination of caring for

Samuel (I was still breast-feeding him at the time) and European travel, I moved into the second trimester with relief. The sickness abated. I enjoyed the new bulge. I bought a few Swedish maternity clothes to accompany me as I grew.

And—I began to feel his movements. The baby tossed and turned inside me and I knew he was there and growing. I felt excited. I felt proud, even. (Two boys! In another time or culture it would have been looked upon as a great achievement to bear two sons.) I allowed myself indulgences I never did with Samuel, being too superstitious: I bought a sweet and superfluous infant outfit, to show the new baby that I was thinking of him and looking forward to meeting him.

I loved him, now, this little fellow. Yes, the news had been a shock, but that was what life was like, wasn't it? We could not always control everything as we hoped, and being a good mother meant being able to adapt to change with some grace.

I was getting ready. I was writing again, and swimming, and taking care of myself. I had weaned Samuel in preparation for the next one's arrival. I was five months pregnant, about twenty-three weeks. When I saw another spot of blood one night, I wasn't even worried. I would call the doctor sometime the next day, just to check in.

⁓

Actually, I forgot. The next morning there was no longer any blood and I pushed the thought aside, moving into my morning routine. It was only when I returned to the house at about lunchtime that it occurred to me that I was having pain. The realization dawned slowly. It was not just pain—it was *that* pain. Yes, it was a contraction. I called the doctor's office and was told to come in. As my own OB was away, I would be seeing a woman who had happened to give me a checkup a few weeks earlier. I remembered her commenting then on my uterine anomaly, "It can mean preterm labor, or a small baby." I did not really understand what was happening. I asked the doctor if I might have to go on bed rest. Yes, I might, but in the meanwhile, what I needed to do was get to the hospital right away.

And then, the proverbial blur. I remember going up to the hospital's third floor, to Labor & Delivery, where I had gone into labor with Samuel (my waters broke at thirty-nine weeks; the baby was breech, and born by Cesarean). I don't know how it happened with Linnaeus. It must have been midday, an innocent time of day, as I walked over from the doctor's office, still very unclear about what was going on. I am not sure when Sedge came to join me. I don't remember being given a room, though I must have been. I did not know or imagine, when I lay down on that bed, that I would not leave the room for another three days. And that I'd leave so much lighter than I had been when I arrived.

The contractions, slow at first, unthreatening, rapidly became more regular and more intense. There must have been hours of them. I don't quite recall the order of events. What I know is that there was a parade of doctors, none of them my familiar beloved Swedish OB, coming in to advise and diagnose. A machine was hooked up to monitor the baby, who was evidently all right, though I was progressing quickly into full-blown labor. I was dilating. A decision was made (by me?

by Sedge? by the two of us together?) to give me drugs to try to slow down the labor. Magnesium. I was told that they were not sure why it worked, but it seemed to, though I should be aware that it had powerful side effects, making the patient nauseous and confused.

I was given magnesium, and became nauseous and confused. For quite a long time (hours? endless minutes?) the drug seemed to have no effect, and the contractions continued, painful, regular. Finally, in the middle of the night, they started to slow down. I drifted into a kind of sleep.

At some point I was seen by a perinatologist who determined that there had been a placental abruption. This meant that the placenta had started to bleed and to tear away from the uterus, and therefore was not going to be able to continue to feed the baby, even if the drugs managed to stop labor. (Usually, in the case of a placental abruption later in a pregnancy, the baby is simply removed immediately. The abruption poses serious health risks to mother and infant both; there's a risk of great blood loss.) The baby might seem all right now, but he could not stay in for long and continue to be nourished. Whether the doctors could in any case stop labor successfully was unclear. I was four or five centimeters dilated already. One OB whom I trusted felt that labor had gone on too long, that the baby would have to be born in the next day or two.

The day and night and day that followed are indeed muddied, though there are encounters I remember and conversations I recall. Samuel came to visit, and it was painful to see him through the tangle of tubes and machines. He seemed cheerful but reluctant to see this alien parent, bedridden and out of reach. Henry had declined to visit me in the hospital so far, fearful perhaps of what he'd find there.

Sedge and I talked. Our son was just under twenty-three weeks old, which at the time was a week or two shy of "viability." One of our visitors was a pregnant doctor who worked on the ward with the preterm babies, who made a forceful case that the term "viability" was, in any case, misleading. She actually told us that she considered the extreme measures taken to try to save some very premature babies' lives to be tantamount to child abuse. She filled us with fear of what would happen to our son if he was born alive and resuscitated in this way: He would be taken from us, wrapped in plastic wrap, put under hot bulbs, given IVs in veins that scarcely existed—he would be more or less physically tormented, in an attempt to "save" his life which would in all likelihood be unsuccessful. She pleaded with us, for his sake, for our family's sake, not to be persuaded to make that attempt.

Another doctor, a perinatologist, told us of the miracles. Some babies of twenty-four weeks had survived. Not every single one was severely compromised in physical and mental health, though most were. They might be deaf or blind, unable to walk, unable to breathe on their own. It was just possible, with drugs, that they might be able to keep the baby inside me until twenty-four weeks. I do remember speaking to this doctor's kind and doubled face (the magnesium affects one's eyesight) and hearing his optimism, hearing his effort to counter the nightmarish image conjured by the other doctor before him. We were visited by Samuel's pediatrician, who told stories of her own experiences watching underinformed parents make the decision to go to dramatic lengths to save their child, thus entering into an unforeseen ordeal that often tore a family apart. She emphasized how hard it could be on the other children in a family, particularly because in the great majority of cases, after weeks or months spent camping out at a hospital, the baby died.

My husband and I listened and talked and, fortunately for us, we arrived at the same understanding based on what we heard. We had a baby boy who had been healthy until now, but he was on his way to entering the world too soon. The placental abruption meant that he was losing his nourishment and might already be too compromised to live, and the labor had progressed to the point that it could not successfully be stopped for long. We did not want to subject our beloved son to the medical establishment's effortful hopes for a miracle. That seemed neither right nor humane to us. If our son was to be born, we wanted him to be born and be with us. We wanted to hold him.

We made the decision, supported by several doctors, to stop the magnesium. I lay in my bed quietly, two days after feeling the first contractions, and waited.

I could still feel my baby boy moving inside me. By this point, we had named him: He was to be called Linnaeus.

⁓

I don't know which part was the most shocking. Was it padding about the room half-naked in the flimsy hospital robe, knowing that the live baby boy within me would soon be dead?

Was it being handed a pamphlet from a trying-to-be-helpful nurse called "Support After Neonatal Death?" with the words "You may not want to look at this now, but hold on to, you'll find it very helpful later"? Or was it simply, basically, the moment in early evening when the contractions began again in earnest, doctors and nurses and my husband clustered around me, and we enacted the classic scene of vaginal delivery (I had not known this with Samuel): *Push, Sylvia, that's right, push, you can do it, breathe, breathe Sylvia, you're doing fine.*

It was that part, of course. That was the most shocking. What was anyone to say when I pushed the little boy out? He weighed a pound. Congratulations were not in order. He was a bundled up, tiny, sweet-faced thing, breathing shallowly, eyes closed, and handed to his father to hold.

It was, soon, a communal scene. By my side, the tearful face of a close friend who had once lost a baby at twenty weeks. Then, a gathering of children. My brother had happened to come over to visit me that evening, just exactly then, with his older son and daughter (they were nine and seven), and Henry had decided to come, too, in the company of a family friend, now that his brother had been born. I was surrounded by people. My brother offered to take a picture of Sedge and me together with little Linnaeus. My niece Grace was holding my hand, her face confused, affectionate, and I made an effort to calm and reassure her, to accept the bewildered goodwill of the people in the room. My nephew Nick held Linnaeus. Henry had a chance to see him. Sedge cradled the bundle lovingly, his face both strong and broken. Afterward, we took much comfort from the fact that for his brief life Linnaeus knew only love and gentleness, and was in a room with his brother and cousins and uncle and parents—a great gathering of family to greet him, and to send him off.

The nurse checked periodically to see whether the baby's heart was still beating. After an hour, it was not. By then, perhaps, the children had gone. I do not remember. Again, there were forms to be filled out. Linnaeus Bell Thomson. Perhaps it was then we checked the box for cremation. The baby was taken away, and I don't remember that, either.

What I do remember is that the room became very quiet. And they got ready to move me. I no longer belonged in Labor & Delivery; I had delivered. I was to be moved for this last night to a different room on a different floor. My sister-in-law generously offered to stay overnight with me there, but after all the noise and drama, and in the aching anticipation of the grief, I knew I wanted to be alone. She helped settle me in, then left. Sometime earlier Sedge had had to return home to be with Samuel.

That other room is still vivid to me, its dark and quiet. There was a view of the city lights from the window. I had asked for something in the way of a spiritual counselor from the hospital, but the awkward man who briefly materialized was unable to offer wisdom or solace. A new series of nurses came to help me, some sensitive, some less so. In one of the many bitter echoes of post-birth ritual, one of them waited for me to produce a quantity of bloody urine. (They always want you to pee afterward, don't they?) Ahead of me was the ordeal of the useless milk coming to my breasts, a painful engorgement, the body's hapless following of its script for new life.

For a while that night I just lay in the quiet, my mind flayed and alert, sleep impossible. The gnawing within had already begun. My belly was not flat yet, of course (I would be asked with a cunning wink, a few weeks later, whether I was happy about my impending arrival, by a man in a hardware store whom I was tempted to violently assault), but it was hollow. I had been emptied. In the days that followed I would keep asking myself how a family that had felt so full before could now feel so terribly impoverished. How could there have opened up in that great fullness an unbearable vacuum?

It was February when we drove up to Lake Tahoe. A calmer time. Months after the cards and flowers and hot meals were over, all the kindnesses of friends that must, eventually, give way to the starkness of regular, unadorned life. It was something to learn how comforting people could be in a time of loss, even when the crisis seems beyond comfort: beautiful notes of sympathy from surprising quarters, a distant cousin or the once-contentious brother. People shelter their graces, often—you don't know about them until the need arises.

We drove up over a long weekend. It's a funny kind of family vacation, a trip that's part fun and frolics in the snow, part ash-scattering. For a day or two we sledded and threw snowballs, and Sedge and Henry climbed the slopes while I watched Samuel tramp and teeter delightedly in the powdery off-white softness. Surreptitiously, while Henry had a skiing lesson, Sedge and I scouted locations for our ritual. We sought a place right by the lake, publicly accessible, and not too far a hike because, as I said nervously, I did not want to have to cope with a meltdown on Henry's part, thanks to too long a walk. Sedge and I were both apprehensive about the emotional event ahead of us.

The morning arrived, and with it new snowfall. After a functional breakfast we took our boots and our box and drove out into the falling flakes to the spot we had chosen.

Henry did have a meltdown, of course. It was inevitable. His boots didn't fit him well and the going wasn't easy and as the adults were emotional, he had every right to be, too. I must have been carrying Samuel, and Sedge, like an Iditarod competitor, tried to mush Henry, get him to keep going, but the boy flagged and failed halfway along and there was a moment when, without brandy or an airlift, it almost seemed as though we would all collapse there in the snow in our raw upset and simply have to wait to be eaten by bears. That, or succumb to hypothermia.

Henry rallied, eventually. Bless him. We made it to our destination: a picnic area by the water, lovely and strange in the thick snow, where we could gather around a barbecue stove for the ritual I had devised. We lit a few candles and placed them on the stove. Sedge and I had each written a few paragraphs for Linnaeus, and Henry a few lines, and we read them out loud to our small frostbitten family before placing the sheets of paper in the flames. Then we gathered the ashes from our words and scattered them, along with the ashes of Linnaeus, under a lone pine by the water's edge. By now

Henry was helping Samuel, holding his hand across the snow and showing him how to take a pinch or two of the fine gray dust to release under our chosen tree. He managed our ritual, and he managed (somehow) to get back to the car, and afterward we were all rewarded with hot cocoas and big platefuls of breakfast at a diner back down the road.

I returned to that place along the lake a couple of years later, in a year when the snowfall had been particularly heavy in the Sierras. I realized that we would not have been able to choose the same spot in a snowier season. I could hardly make it out there for my solo pilgrimage. While a friend waited with Samuel and Romilly in the car—our daughter was nearly one, born a year and a half after Linnaeus died—I tramped along an obscure, snow-thickened path, the same two or three hundred yards that had previously caused us so much difficulty.

As I walked I could hardly locate the barbecue area. The snow was as high as the tops of the picnic tables. I was walking across it precariously to find our place, and though tears starred my vision, making the landscape doubly unfamiliar, I did find it. There was our tree—Linnaeus's tree. I watched the water and the mountains, the mauves and blues and slates, the air and waves. We did choose a beautiful place for him, and that was comforting. We had done our best, in the end.

Three of the five of us remember Linnaeus. Once, from a plane flying over the Sierras, Henry looked down toward the lake and mentioned him. He has drawn pictures of Linnaeus and commemorated him with Sedge and me. (Not long ago,

Henry asked me what I thought it would be like now if Linnaeus were alive and I made him laugh by saying, "Can you imagine how he and Samuel would fight over their toys?") The other two, the little ones, don't yet know about him. He is the ghost between them, between brother and sister; a shadow sibling. A might-have-been. He was an hour, and a light, and a gift. We miss him still.

On Desire: A Conversation Between Husband and Wife

Julianna Baggott and David Scott

From Julianna to David

I can hear people whispering that we've taken more than our share—as if children were our sustenance and we're fattened already and still thinking about lapping at the buffet for a fourth time. And on my last trip to the city to visit my lifelong girlfriends, New Yorkers for a decade now and all childless, I sensed a feeling of starvation, a desperation among them like that of the Great Depression. If I talk of our three kids, even casually, the room churns with emotion. They've rocketed through their careers and are now all eyeing motherhood. There was a time when they observed my babies the way one would a homemade art project—a cocked head, an *oh-that's-nice*. But things have changed. The air is filled not so much with jealousy, but wanting.

Do you and I have a great hunger? Do we want too much? Is our desire to have a big family a kind of weakness? And what is our hunger really about? Isn't desire the flip side of fear? We've both confessed that we're afraid of the way the world demands that we hand our children over. The more children we have the more we have to fear. Does fear work this way? Is it exponential? And not only fear. Deciding to have another child is saying yes to more—more joy, more grief, more love, confusion, noise . . .

And, the truth is, the fear begins now. We already have four children, including the one we lost. I don't tell you how he still exists. He's a boy, tall, thin, with twisted legs—a quiet observer. He's five years old now. In August, I feel the emptiness of a birthday that has no birth date.

For two people who tell each other everything, who've been talking nonstop for thirteen years, we don't linger here. Maybe we should linger here.

From David to Julianna

Here's where I linger: you've told me it's my turn to write, so I sit with the laptop on my thighs and begin to settle in when the door opens. It's you, the great love of my life, my desire, my leg, my nourishment. What's that? I can't quite make it out because of your sudden laryngitis. You look like you're scolding me. "My God," you whisper, "don't put that thing on your lap. They say it causes infertility."

I love the way you protect me, and by protecting me, are trying to give me more. You shake your head at our friends who've been snipped. The vasectomy—the great end of possibilities. What if, you say, I die, and your new wife has never had a child and wants to have children with you. See how you're always giving to me, even in your imagined death.

Death has come to us before. Your great-aunts, my

grandfather who I barely knew, the neighbor girl who died in a sledding accident, and our friend Betsy who you found curled toward the handgun. We have loved our way through all this sadness.

And the baby . . . he was mine, too. (Here, I'm lingering.) As if the blackness on the ultrasound screen was something that could so easily be taken away, but it wasn't. I had to call your father and tell him. I said, "This baby didn't make it." And for the first time, I had truly and irreversibly failed a child. What hadn't I done right? How could I have forgotten to help you: vitamins, exercise, vegetables? How could I have given you the wrong seed? I wish I hadn't—for all the pain it caused you, caused both of us.

And still, here I am, cocked for you. Aiming at you what has become (not to sound too melodramatic but . . .) a dangerous weapon. I want more, in the face of what I know. It's not money or stuff. It's not the diapers or the sleeplessness or the pride in that first step. (Since I've been the one at home among the chaos of kids for years now, I'm not saying any of this with a blind eye to the reality of child rearing.) It's more of you that I want. One more angle, one more topic of conversation, one more knowing sigh we share in the day before we both fall asleep.

You're waving at me now, across the room, your voice only guttural and shushing. Don't speak. Get your voice back. I want to talk to you about the possibility of another baby and the one we lost. Remember that wedding we went to, where the mother of the groom said she was meant to have more children—and she'd had six boys? We've wondered about that statement for years. I feel meant to have another child, I feel meant for the dizzying complexity that kid will bring.

From Julianna to David

It was a miscarriage, and I was the carriage. I imagine myself rattling over cobblestone, a wobbly thing on wooden wheels. It wasn't your fault. I can tell you that as easily as you can tell me the same. Still, I feel sorry for you. I got to hold the child inside of me, and you never did. I don't think it makes logical sense. I was nauseous, slack with fatigue. I never got to feel him kick—just a few weeks shy. But still it seems like a gift to have been able to carry the baby with me, if only for a short time.

I am afraid. So many things wind back to the pain of losing the baby. I wound myself to Betsy's body. I knew that her daughters were at camp, that John was away on business, and when I saw her newspapers still on the stoop in the evening, I was well aware that she might already be gone. The thought had presented itself: She'd tried to kill herself before so it was always possible, more than possible, maybe even inevitable. (We knew the risk when we became friends with her—she had always been open about her suicidal desires and her previous attempt—but knowing the risks doesn't help prepare us for loss.) After I found her stiff body, bluish, and after I'd called 911, I was hysterical. I cried out Betsy, my baby. My baby, Betsy. Loss is loss is loss. It will find a harmony inside of memory—and pull it up more sharply. Loss resounds. It collects and magnifies. One loss calling to another and another.

From David to Julianna

Good God, the ache of it makes me stand and pace, even now. (Betsy is an ache we wish to rub down—and down and down—until the ache stops.) You cannot be sorry for me, sweet love. I'm only the beggar here. You've given me time and these children I haven't deserved. I'd been raised to believe that love was a resource, that after you gulped it, it might be gone. You've helped me to understand that the main property of love is that it ramifies, expands to meet need. This is not a quality reserved for loss.

But I am supposed to be lingering still. It was dark. We had no idea if you'd be able to have another. And the technician in the imaging center handled it all so badly. I hated the way you moaned, the sob echoing from the black stain on the screen. "Is that the baby?" I asked the stupefied tech.

"Yes," she said, extremely unsure. And then she left.

"What's the matter?" I asked. "What is it?"

But you already knew, knew in a way that I couldn't, in which dread precedes devastating news, the way a phone ringing at the wrong time of night is never good.

Then there was the sterile hour I spent while you were having the D and C done. I think I read about sports or some dry *New Yorker* short story where the characters obsessed over the dry fabric of a tablecloth and left a lip stain on their cup of green tea. I never felt farther away from you. I looked around the waiting room. Old men turned inward, women my mother's age knitting some fabric amid idle chatter. The news prattling on in high spirits. I didn't know that what would come next would be a flood of miscarriage stories. It

seemed like everyone I knew could tell at least two miscarriage stories: mothers, daughters, children, wives, teachers.
The world of miscarriage was a secret society we'd joined by
accident, by living.

From Julianna to David
And afterward, how you tore up the bathroom tiles, went
rummaging through the house's piping for a leak. You worked
and worked, trying to make something right. (I do not want
to join more secret societies. How many are there? I sense
them everywhere.)

From David to Julianna
And then, how you tore into your first novel, a beautiful
frenzy. You wrote and wrote. And I kept saying, "Write,
write," and I watched you at the door to your office lost in
it, and I wanted to come in, and I wanted to leave you
alone. The main metaphor in that first novel was drowning,
and I wanted to wrap you in a yellow flotation jacket and
bring you back up, through the murk. But I'm certain it was
clear at the bottom during those months. So I often left you
to it.

(The secret societies will keep coming. I'm sorry, but it's
true. No one wants to join the society of survivors. Survivors
of suicide was another, but for us there was no choice. I've
left you alone with that as well. I try to hold you up as much
as I can. I want to take these losses away from you. I want to
be a thief, with a specialty in loss, and one who refuses to
give things back, even when caught red-handed.)

From Julianna to David

You are no thief. You wouldn't really steal our losses, because you know that the losses are what have come to make up my constitution. One day our constitutions will be all that's left of us. (I love your constitution.) I think our constitutions will age well together.

Today, thanks to my laryngitis I can only whisper at you, at the kids. I've taught them all which clapping rhythm equals their name—one clap for Phoebe, two for Finneas, three for Theo, one slow and two fast for the neighbor kid visiting. Fast, urgent clapping—by the way—means *you*, that I need you now. And when I whisper, the kids whisper back. It's natural to forget my laryngitis and to assume for a moment that someone is sleeping somewhere nearby—a sleeping baby, a boy we refuse to forget—one that grows up alongside the others—a baby not yet conceived.

My Others

Miranda Field

What happens is the child I'm waiting for dies inside me, but I continue to carry it. I'm pregnant with the dead child for another three weeks. The pregnancy falls quiet around the twelfth week, and this is a relief. I don't know the quiet child is dead. I'm happy no longer to be feeling sick. I'm like the self-absorbed stranger at the bar or in the train car, who keeps talking on and on after the one he's talking to has gotten up and left.

I fall through many floors of silence. During the cab ride to the hospital, the tense, nervous silence between Tom and me, prelude to the technician's professional silence during the sonogram, then that of the summoned doctor. The baby's lack of vital signs, its diminutive size—all wrong for a fetus in its fourth month of gestation, like a small beach pebble—its utter stillness. The zero-sum click of the door as the chicken-hearted doctor escapes. It's the technician who speaks up, so I can finally hit the ground. My mind is forced to take in the fact: "The fetus is nonviable." Still, my witless body doesn't grasp what's happened. It continues to be pregnant. It holds tight the body of the dead child as if it believes it might yet come to term. I have to hail another cab, go home, call the clinic whose number the midwife quietly scribbles for me on the back of a prescription pad. I have to make arrangements for the medical termination of this pregnancy my body still believes in.

$\sim$

Almost twenty years before this, I went to a clinic to arrange for an abortion. It's not something I ever talk about. It was in London, where I grew up, and during a terrible time in my life. I was fifteen, lost, my family in pieces, my life a disaster. The doctor who performed the abortion, at a National Health hospital, called me a whore. Actually, he called me a "trollop." Who uses that word? This was 1977, not 1877. Nevertheless, I knew what it meant. "If you were my daughter," he said, "I'd put you over my knee." He said this while he was examining my breasts. They were swollen, tender, with eerily vivid blue veins fanning out from the darkened nipples. Already my body had changed. I had thrown up that morning, out the window of the car, stuck in heavy traffic, as my mother took me to the hospital. I'd almost passed out the previous week, at school, in an early-morning physics class. I wanted to fast-forward past this time in my life, for it to be over with. I wanted to be unconscious, asleep, to wake up again somewhere else, *as* someone else. I remember surfacing from the general anesthetic after the procedure in a cold hospital bed, a tired-voiced Jamaican nurse chiding me not to cry. I didn't realize I was crying. I was crying in my sleep, but

I woke up hearing someone else, another one of the younger patients, crying in a bed near mine. When I finally got out of bed, on wobbly legs, to use the bathroom, I remember the flooding—bright red splotches of blood on the bathroom floor. I leaned against the tile wall, nauseous and dizzy, and sobbed like a child, my childhood done.

⁓

I ask my midwife if it would be possible to just wait a little. Let the miscarriage proceed naturally, unfold by itself (or let it not—my frantic, irrational hope that this is all a mistake, that if I wait, maybe the baby will wake up, start to grow again). "If you don't go to the clinic within the next couple of days," she tells me, "you'll end up in the emergency room this weekend, hemorrhaging." This is a Thursday. I don't even have a day to think, to let the truth settle in. I make the appointment. And I'm a terrified adolescent again, walking up the few steps to the clinic's entrance. It's a seedy place, with shabby plastic chairs, worn carpeting, sickly lighting. In the waiting room, there are two young girls. Three young boys. A television is on, sound turned down low, a horrible soap opera. Why does television always continue to prattle on through all catastrophes?

Two weeks after the D and C, I sit surrounded by pregnant women, waiting to see my midwife for a post-op examination. I feel indescribably wrong in the presence of all these hugely rounded bellies. Defunct. Defective. I sit in the waiting room staring at a poster of an enormous open-throated orchid in watercolor pinks and peach and lavender. I've stared at it so many times before I almost could paint it from memory. This is the room where my first pregnancy, as mysterious and abstract as it was in the early weeks and months, unfolded exactly as the books and charts predicted—until, in the last stages, the pregnancy manifested beyond doubt, my child's life a certainty. Now, as I sit, finding it harder by the minute to hold back my tears, I hear, billowing from one of the examining rooms, a baby's amplified heartbeat, unmistakable, an astounding, speedy, subaquatic sound that breaks me. "It's nothing you did or didn't do," I'm told, when the midwife finally sees me. "It's just a mistake of nature. These things happen." No one seems to want to let me feel a part of the root cause of this event. They insist on its randomness. But it's almost a relief, a temporary cure, literally—the way an aspirin is for a headache—to be able to blame something, even if there's nothing to blame but my body.

The feeling of emptiness that the pregnancy's evaporation has left me with brings me close to a perpetual state of panic. My midwife claims my system is slowly returning to "normal," to its non-pregnant state. I want to stop this return. I want to be pregnant again, immediately, as if that would stop inexorable events, reverse the pregnancy's collapse. I'm cautioned to wait until my hormones have "settled down," till I've had at least two normal menstrual cycles, before Tom and I try to conceive again. However, though the information sheet from the clinic where my D and C was performed tells me to expect my periods to return in four to seven weeks, after several endlessly long months I still haven't bled. I wait, but not patiently. I wait the way an animal waits to be let out of a room.

I can't stop working at the door, though nothing gives. Every time I pee, every time I shower, every time I feel the vaguest hint of a distant, distant shadow of a cramp, I rush to the bathroom to look for blood. Nothing. All I want is that one sign that everything's okay. It doesn't seem too much to ask. But my body has shut down, stopped communicating.

Months pass and I wait for the green light, for the bio-chemical signal that says I'm fit to conceive again, for the go-ahead from my practitioner. I fixate on the medical facts, as if they're simply there to be overcome, as if I have control over them; I focus on the biological hurdles, as if they're everything. But, truly, it's not my physical self that's lost in this fiction, that can't recover.

Even Tom—my husband, my love, my closest-ever friend, my lost baby's father—can't quite know how I feel, can't reach me where I've gone. The therapist I see, at Tom's urg-ing, waits a long while for me to say something, and then, when I can't find a single thing to say, asks what my silence would say if it could speak. Nothing. Such intensely private fixation on a loved one who is and always was invisible, un-verifiable; so much unexplained, strange mourning behavior in the absence of a funeral. All this makes the mother griev-ing for her unborn child seem a little deranged to the world that keeps looking away, pretending nothing's happened, or otherwise claims over and over it *wishes* it could understand. I want to feel my baby start to move when what would have been my fifth month begins. When my baby's due date arrives I'm sick with wanting the body weight of my baby in my arms. When you miscarry after a previous birth, the mass of that absent body is excruciatingly palpable. Four years earlier, I'd felt my first child somersault inside me. I touched his impossibly tender, birth-bruised flesh, his hot, downy infant head. I stared, traced with my finger, photographed—with that fanatical, self-abandoning fixation of new motherhood—the whorls and feathery patterns of his hair slicked to his skull after his passage through me. I've followed, since, his slow unfolding into unimaginable complexity. At this point, if I were a figure in a myth, a draft of something metaphysical and merciful might be offered to help me forget my longing. I could ask for pharmaceuticals to do the same, but I don't want to let my longing go.

The miscarriage happens in October. We've already announced the pregnancy to friends and family, to casual acquaintances, to the man in the dry cleaner's. Now, as months go by, and in my distraction I grow thinner and thinner, the privacy I bury myself in like a winter coat restricts my movements. The unspoken is increasingly and awkwardly obvious. The year is winding down, the parks and gardens going dormant, but not the city itself. In a way the city's just waking up in the fall, is most full of life in winter. I'm busy—that is, I *look* busy; work is frantic. But inside, I'm experiencing a kind of implosion, in slow motion and silent and completely possessing. Parties and gatherings have become impossible for me to endure. I stay home as much as I can. I'm glad when the weather dips below zero and automatically cancels all my social obligations.

Psychoanalyst Adam Philips writes, in *The Beast in the Nursery*, "Tell me what makes you enraged—what makes you feel truly diminished—and I will tell you what you believe or what you want to believe about yourself." Pregnant with my first son, I grew huge in every way, very quickly—fat and happy—on the discovery that I could give life, and sustain it, cause it to grow. One aspect of miscarriage that's seldom discussed is what happens when a suddenly supercharged sense of self-confidence is precipitously reversed. How it can hit the woman with a shocking, vertiginous crisis of identity. Miscarriage does this to me, deals me something of an existential blow. When I became a mother for the first time, and found my milk flowed whenever my baby cried, my body had seemed miraculous to me. In the aftermath of my miscarriage, I feel about myself, my body, as one feels passing through an intersection on a highway where a fatality has happened. The physical space itself feels fundamentally desolate, intrinsically linked with death.

⁓

This morning I carry a brown paper lunch sack filled with technical problems to the hardware store. The clerk and I sit on the floor in a corner unscrewing splinter-sized screws with elfin Phillips-head screwdrivers, testing connections, fitting sequin-sized washers and wing-nuts in place. The problem we eventually root out is one loose wire in a tiny motor meant to make a rainbow-checkered disc revolve, magic-lantern style, above a miniature bulb—the brain inside my children's psychedelic, fiber-optic haunted Halloween house. Now I pull from my bag a fire engine that was really a vibrating tooth-brush whose lights have quit flashing, now a pumpkin night-light, and a plastic creature and its snapped off tail. These are a child's valuables, objects of unfathomable private passions.

Giving birth for the first time changed me radically, at the level of what I can only call my soul, though I wish I had a better word for it. I wish I had another word for what makes me keep track of all these endless fragments of all these bro-ken magical gadgets, and buy so many kinds of glue, and work so tirelessly to put the pieces back together. For why I sense the secret potential of every viable rubber band on the side-walk. There's nothing in the Pregnancy and Birth section of the bookstore that speaks to how your focus alters, your per-spectives shift. Biological explication and practical advice fill those shelves, demystifying pregnancy and birth, for good and obvious reasons. And discipline and nutrition advice fills the Parenting shelves. But, no matter how much birth is ra-tionalized, the mystery doesn't go away. I gave birth, some-thing filled me (something scary and beautiful, exhausting, unmanageable, transformative), and I felt as though I'd carry it inside forever—a sense of repletion, of being perilously overfilled at times, but full. The overwhelming aspects of birth and new motherhood are undeniable. The always ongo-ing, nonnegotiable tasks of infant care can seem surreal in their demands. But daily life with my infant was also sensu-ally and emotionally supersaturated, exhausting but gratify-ing. My mind was groggy from lost sleep, but aspects of my mental life, too, were more wide awake, more existentially at-tuned than ever before. While my baby slept and I refused to heed the constantly repeated advice to nap myself, I wrote the poems that would become my first book. If I sound like the cat that ate the canary, I guess it's how I felt.

Now, in the parallel universe of solitude and silence following the miscarriage, I'm unbearably empty. My beloved four-year-old is a helpless bystander. After the abortion, years earlier, I'd spiraled down into a terrible, perplexing, and long-lasting depression, farther and farther away from my difficult but familiar place in the world. That's another story. It is and isn't part of this one. This time, I have a working life to maintain, and a marriage, and a living child. I keep myself afloat through an elaborate tightrope act of magical thinking. It goes like this: If I can conceive another, more hospitable body for my baby to inhabit, if I make it well and quickly, I might coax it back.

What was this *it*? I've mentioned that the concept of a "soul," distinct and separate from the body, doesn't sit easily with me. But in extremity, it's what I fixed upon: that elusive but specific essence of my child. I hold this secret plan inside: I won't try for another baby. I'll capture *this* one again. I get fanatical, and a kind of panic consumes me when this plan takes hold, as if I'm driven to possess one specific firefly that's slipped through a tear in my net, and none other out of all the flickering swarm will do. If I don't mend the net fast enough, it will be too late, it will disappear, lost in darkness. But the midwife cautions me to bide my time: You don't want to put yourself through this all over again.

I wake up in a panic in the black middle of the night, several weeks after the miscarriage, recalling the clinic's Pine-Sol smell, the face of the anesthetist telling me to count backward from ten to nothing, the curious, useless paper shoes I'd woken up wearing in the recovery room. Then it hits, in the middle of all these shaken-loose details, the sudden realization that my child's body (and it *was* a body, though no one ever said that word, only "matter" and "tissue," rendered shapeless, ungraspable) had simply been discarded along with all the clinic's "medical waste" of that day. On a pregnancy-loss website someone referred me to, I'd read accounts of ceremonies, funerals, ritualized good-byes. But it was too late for me to say good-bye. I'd not had the presence of mind to ask for my child's remains to be returned to me. As I lie there, I remember the doctor warning me of heavy bleeding for a week or more. I remember the awful quantity of blood, years before, on the hospital floor, when I'd sobbed for my damaged self. But this time, I'd bled lightly, for only a few days. Was what I'd lost so substanceless?

I trawl the Internet to find a book I'd thumbed through one afternoon, years earlier, while I was working my way through graduate school in a bookstore. It's a photo essay I'm looking for, whose title I can't remember, though I've never forgotten the power the subject held for me. I Google "garden," and "miscarriage" and "abortion," but I don't find what I'm looking for. The book was about a garden in Japan where unborn children are remembered—stillbirths and miscarriages as well as abortions. The garden is filled to the brim with homemade paper dolls, hundreds and hundreds and hundreds of them, all different, like brightly colored pinwheels, fluttering in the breeze. On each doll is written a message or prayer. How unthinkable is such a place here, now, in the United States. What a political battleground would such a garden be. In America, you can't mourn an aborted child. The woman who miscarries and the woman who voluntarily aborts are placed in separate categories. To speak of grief in the context of abortion (with or without second thoughts) is to risk aligning yourself with those who call themselves "prolife," who would reduce infinite complexities of circumstance and emotion to simple abstractions. Even the thought of such a place existing today, in the United States, seems dangerous. But the memory garden for miscarried, stillborn and aborted children (in a province just outside Kyoto, I think), is filled not with explanations or justifications, not with politics or polemics, but with private missives written on the folds of fluttering paper sleeves, by women, men, mothers, fathers. No one's story, no one's account of grief or sorrow or relief is questioned or held to account.

⁓

"Every birth is also a death," says poet Gillian Conoley. I've undergone the transformation she speaks of: the "split of the body" and psychic deepening that follows labor's "journey to the void and back." Much of what you've known of yourself, and both known and imagined of your unborn child, is demolished in the process of birth. But if pregnancy leading to motherhood first breaks you open, then opens you to a larger life, pregnancy ending in a death just leaves you broken. The puzzle you're left with is how to assimilate this turn of events: the death of someone who never lived but was all in your imagination; who was real, and who opened up an enormous space inside you, but will never fill it. The world you discover in the aftermath of miscarriage seems so impossibly empty.

~

I hear a story on the local news channel sometime that fall, about a woman whose child was abducted from a playground while she turned her back for a few minutes, forgot to watch, became engrossed in some mother-to-mother conversation. If a child can slip from your own body, of course a child can slip from a playground. From any place. In November, as the nights grow longer, colder, we bring our four-year-old into bed with us, where I watch him all night long. He comes down with croup twice that winter, waking up gasping in the darkness for breath. The first time, we don't know what's happening. I'm certain I'm holding my dying child. The second time, we close the bathroom window and door, as we've been taught, turn the shower on hot, until the steam is so dense you can't see through it, and the room becomes a rain forest. I hold him in my arms in the steam, rocking, rocking, saying his name, stroking his back until his screaming stops, his rigid body softens, his breath comes back. In the playground, all that winter and spring, I shadow him so closely he complains. I hold his hand too insistently wherever we go.

⟞⟋

"The baby's gone away," I tell my son Willie one morning, when it's no longer okay to just say nothing. He presses me: "Where's it gone?" I, ever the vaguely spiritual agnostic, tell him something like: "Back into nature, in the air and clouds and leaves." And as I say it, I believe it. But when he cries so hard and long it frightens me, I take it back. I say: "But not forever."

⟞⟋

My second pregnancy loss was different from my first. I wanted this child. But both losses have haunted me. In the case of the abortion, the imagined child does exist, does linger, but fades more quickly. In the case of the miscarriage, I can't let go. I persist in denying the finality of death, plotting to redo what's been undone, until, sometime early in spring, I'm stunned to find I'm pregnant again. I'm incredibly lucky, able to conceive effortlessly again, once my body has recovered. But nothing is taken for granted this time. I go forward with trepidation. Many superstitious personal rituals (delaying the choosing of a name, not mentioning too soon the secret which, if brought to light, might disappear) carry me along till my second son, Finnian, is born.

Each time I visit a new gynecologist (vicissitudes of HMOs), I answer the routine questions: number of pregnancies—four; number of births—two. The question, the imbalanced equation, which the gynecologist jots down in shorthand figures and symbols, always sends a tiny shock through me. Makes me think of the disparity between my two crazy, amazing children, and my other two, the phantom siblings. How full, how exponentially more noisy and chaotic and enriched my household, my life, and my living children's lives might have been with them here. And then I wonder what their own lives might have been—the lives of my "others."

Part of me still thinks of the unborn child who disappeared, the fugitive who left me frantic, who made me the mother of a missing child, as the same one who eventually came home with me and, this time, stayed. For Willie, Finn, Tom, and me, this has become one of those eccentricities of personal history that families uncritically keep around, fact mixed with fiction, spoken in a private language, in private space. "Finnian always changes his mind, Mom," Willie will say. "Remember when he came, then went away, then came back again?" Of my first lost child, I seldom think, and never speak.

I have no idea when the first child I carried might have been born. But every spring since the miscarriage, there's a stretch on the calendar I don't like to look at, a missing birthday I'm still aware of. The baby I miscarried, who was supposed to come when the trees were all in blossom, made way for Finnian. My second son comes to us in the late fall, a whole other season. By the time he wakes up from his birth drowse and begins to register the world around him, it's already freezing. It turns into a winter of incredible blizzards.

My children are so transparent at times, I have to pretend I don't see through their disguises, their ruses and secrets. (Finnian loves to "hide" from us after his bath—stark naked, in the middle of the living room—by shutting his eyes and burying his head in his arms.) But they change so constantly, so suddenly, in ways impossible to anticipate. Whole regions of their lives are perfect ciphers. Soon after Finnian's birth— moments after—in November twilight, Willie climbs onto the hospital bed, puts his head on my breast, pushes his face into the warm space between me and the tiny, red, wrinkled face of his brother, and whispers something very quietly, very privately, into the newborn ear. I don't catch what he says. It's not intended for me.

Are You Still Three?

Elizabeth Oness

When our son was two years old, blue-eyed and preco-
cious, strangers started telling me it was time to have
another baby. At the post office, at the grocery store, women
would wag their fingers at my smiling son and say, "He needs
a little sister." I'd smile politely and think they didn't know
what the hell they were talking about.

I did want another child, or part of me did, but I was tired,
physically and mentally, of juggling household logistics and
childcare with my husband. We had just finished our PhDs
without putting our son in day care. We took our comprehen-
sive exams when Jensen was eleven months old, and during
my son's first year, my two repeated questions were "Could he
be hungry again?" and "Where's the Norton anthology?" Our
study schedules revolved around Jensen's sleep (or lack of
sleep) and nursing. Day care was the obvious solution, but I
didn't want to leave Jensen with anyone I didn't know, and
didn't want him to get sick. Sleep, in those years, seemed more
precious than money, which we had very little of, and our
schedules were so delicately arranged that a sick child would

throw everything into disarray. We did have two friends who would watch Jensen for an afternoon, and those windows of uninterrupted time seemed an unbelievable luxury.

Motherhood was consuming, but right after my husband landed a tenure-track job in La Crosse, Wisconsin, we decided to have another child. Of course, I weighed it all: another baby, more insanity, more distraction, less sleep. I felt anxious about the idea that a second child would cut further into my writing time, but decided this was the time to do it, since life with a two-year-old was already full of upheaval.

I was pregnant twice after Jensen was born, when he was two and a half, and when he turned three. Both times, I passed the "safe" twelve-week mark before losing the pregnancy.

During my pregnancies, I tried to do everything right: filtered water, organic food, green cleaners, no caffeine. Without coffee, I felt fuzzy and inarticulate, as if my personality had been erased. Friends told me, "Oh, I drank coffee when I was pregnant, it's fine," but a vestigial Catholic guilt rose up in me, and I didn't want to do anything to hurt the baby. Once or twice a week, I would make a cup of tea and leave it steeping on the counter. The longer it steeped, the more I wanted it, and the more I wanted it, the more I felt I shouldn't have it. This charade was neurotic; I knew it. About half of the time I poured the tea out, the other half I drank it, and nothing ever tasted so good in my life.

I had my first miscarriage at home, on the night before my husband's thirty-fourth birthday. Chad spent most of the following day at the hospital with me. I tried to think of the miscarriage as a temporary setback, and let myself be comforted by the fact that I had a child who still liked to be cuddled and held.

When I asked the midwife how long I should wait before getting pregnant again, she told me that I didn't need to wait—after one period I could get pregnant again. Later, searching medical studies on the web, I learned that when a woman gets pregnant within three months of a miscarriage, there's a significantly higher rate of her having another miscarriage or problem pregnancy. I wish someone had told me this. I would have waited, let my body gain a bit more strength—or would I? I didn't question whether it was the right thing to do. Like many women after a miscarriage, I wanted to get pregnant again, right away. And so I did.

~

This time, I didn't walk around on eggshells, but I didn't announce my pregnancy, either. I'd made it through the first trimester before and, superstitious, I didn't want to tempt fate.

I lost the third pregnancy at sixteen weeks, a little girl with a profound genetic abnormality. The doctors said it was nothing I'd done. I was older; my eggs were older. It was simply bad luck. Still, I felt that something was terribly wrong—in the cosmic sense—that this should happen again.

~

When we moved to Wisconsin, my husband and I started seeing an acupuncturist for routine things, such as back pain from sitting at the computer. Tune-ups, one might say. But acupuncture isn't routinely used on pregnant women, and

I hadn't seen the acupuncturist in a while, with two pregnancies in quick succession.

It felt comforting to go to his office, which was scented with the tang of Chinese herbs. I told him what had happened since I'd last seen him. He took my pulse, looked at my tongue and eyes, and it didn't take him long to arrive at his diagnosis.

He explained in Chinese terms, and when I looked at him doubtfully he paraphrased. "When you get pregnant and you're worn down, you tend to have a pregnancy like this, the sort of condition where the lights are on, but no one's home."

I looked out the window, at the wedge of parking lot in my line of vision. He started again, reminding me of how frenetic the past few years had been.

"You and your husband did academic job searches while taking care of a toddler. You flew around the country for days-long interviews. You sold one house and bought another, and moved all your possessions from Missouri to Wisconsin. And now you're taking care of a two-year-old while your husband is working. So you were exhausted, but you decided to get pregnant. You had a miscarriage, and instead of waiting, you got pregnant again. The classical Chinese literature suggests that women have babies five years apart. I'm not saying that's necessary, but it suggests that a woman's body needs time to build itself up between pregnancies. In Chinese medical terms, we say: There's not enough blood to anchor a spirit. Not physical blood, but a deficiency of chi."

He said this more gently than I'm recording it here. His tone was not admonishing, but his reasoning had the hammer-fall of truth.

The acupuncturist's diagnosis didn't contradict what the Western doctors had said. It was simply put in different terms. I'd gotten pregnant when I was exhausted and this was the result. I thought of all the people I knew who'd had healthy children close together. My mother was thirty-one when I was born, and she had my sister Patty seventeen months after I was delivered. As a child, Patty was bigger, more athletic, and more social than I was. Patty has two daughters who are fifteen months apart, and her second child is lovely and healthy as well. So why did this happen to me?

Driving home, it occurred to me that I hadn't truly asked myself whether I should get pregnant, or whether it was the right time to do it. I loved being a mother, so I weighed the logistical problems against the idea of another cuddly infant. Instead of thinking about getting pregnant in a spiritual sense, I'd considered it merely in terms of the chaos quotient: Life is chaotic already, why not do it now? Perhaps for something as important as having a child, I should have been a bit more attuned, considered the matter a bit more deeply.

The acupuncturist, Terry, had given me some direct instructions. I needed to buy medicinal Chinese herbs and cook them into chicken soup, the kind made from an actual chicken carcass, to strengthen my system. I should use a moxa box, a small, round device about five inches in diameter, on my stomach several times a week. It was supposed to strengthen my chi. And most important, I should not get pregnant for at least one year. I must have looked at him aghast. I was thirty-eight. If I waited another year, I'd be delivering a baby when I was forty.

Terry ordered eight different packages of Chinese herbs for me to cook into the soup. The Shan yao was chalky white. Some of the herbs looked like dried berries, others like bark or roots or sticks. I still have the recipe:

3 medium pieces	Dang shen	(*Codonopsis* root)
5 pieces	Jujube	(red date)
6 to 8 pieces	Long yan	(Longan fruit)
30 pieces	Gou qi zi	(Lycium fruit)
3 pieces	Shan yao	(*Dioscorea* root)
1 piece	Bai zhu	(*Atractylodes*)
3 pieces	Bai shao yao	(white peony root)
1 large piece	Dang gui pian	(*Angelica sinensis*)

During the simmering, the Long yan, which resembled a walnut, cracked open to reveal a gellied, seaweed-like substance. The jujubes were sweet, like currants. After cooking, I was to strain out the herbs and drink some broth, every day, to build up my strength.

So I made chicken soup and drank it faithfully. I took vitamins. I used the moxa box, which was comforting, like lying down with a hot-water bottle. And I promised that I wouldn't even think about whether to get pregnant again.

But standing at the sink one night, washing dishes, I had a crushing realization: If I waited another six months to get pregnant, as my acupuncturist suggested, and everything went fine, the baby would arrive just as Jensen was starting kindergarten. Just when life was starting to become normal, when I'd have more time to write, we'd be back to diapers, strollers, high chairs, worrying about immunizations, choking, the general disasters of the world. I felt stunned. I don't know why this hadn't occurred to me before, and I counted the months again just to make sure. Yes, if I waited, and everything went like clockwork, I'd be starting all over again just as I was starting to get free.

I told myself that I could be more brave and optimistic, more spiritually centered with the next baby. But the genetic problems with my last pregnancy frightened me, and my desire to have another child didn't outweigh my fear of calamity. And that was it. I realized that if I couldn't conceive a child while feeling a certain measure of happiness and optimism, it simply wasn't the right thing to do.

When I told Chad what I felt, he took it in without saying much. I believe he felt some of the same ambivalence I did: relieved on one hand, sad on the other. I knew he wanted a daughter as well as a son, although he was careful not to say so in those years, not wanting to give me more to worry over. We both would have liked a house that felt full. In general, we tend to think of family happiness as crowded and abundant. All those Kodak commercials, all those advertisements, are filled with families of two children—a boy and a girl.

❦

My husband and I run a literary fine press, and in that time of pregnancy and miscarriage, some of my correspondence fell through the cracks due to sheer fatigue. I had owed a response to a poet for a long time, and when I finally wrote to him, apologizing for my long silence, I explained that I'd been pregnant, and not, then pregnant again, then not. Months later, when I called him on the phone for some advice, he asked, "Are you still three?" Sitting in my office, looking out over the backyard littered with fallen leaves, I thought that his question was deft and thoughtful, one of the kindest ways that anyone had asked.

We are still three. And I have this to report: We are just fine. More than fine, we're happy, when not coping with life's vicissitudes. I don't feel regret about choosing not to get pregnant again. My sisters have had children in the last few years, and my nieces and nephews are adorable, but they don't make me want to roll the dice again.

As three, we've done things that we probably wouldn't have taken on if Jensen had a sibling who was five years younger. I don't mean to suggest that these activities are preferable to having a child, only that certain things have been fun that otherwise might have been stressful.

We often spend part of the summer on the road to sell our press's books. One summer, when Jensen turned eight, we called on universities throughout the Southeast. At night, we went to minor-league baseball games. After a day of driving, finding our way around campus, unpacking in yet another hotel, it was fun to sit outside, eat ice cream, and watch a game. That summer, we saw the Louisville Bats, the Lexington Kings, the Nashville Sounds, the Rome Braves, the Greensboro Bats, the Carolina Mudcats, the Danville Braves, the Williamsport Crosscutters, the Buffalo Bison, and the Toledo Mudhens (twice). If we'd had a two- or three-year-old exploring the dirty cement, threatening meltdown due to the late hours or lack of a nap, it would have been aggravating rather than fun. This is not to say that a few minor-league games make up for a child that might have been, but we've done things as a family of three that we've all enjoyed. Jensen calls our old Ford Aerostar van our "traveling fort," and sometimes, while on our long drives, I feel as if our lives are contained, that I have all that is most precious in the world with me.

Being pregnant allowed me not to make any big plans for several years, but in the aftermath of those lost pregnancies, there was a sudden opening: What did I want? One thing I wanted was a sense of community. We'd made some wonderful friends in La Crosse, but I was mainly identified as a faculty wife. When Chad introduced me to people and told them I was a writer, they would smile sympathetically, glance at my son and say, "Oh, how nice that you have a hobby." So I went on the job market and found a tenure-track job. Chad left his job to spend more time printing books and fathering.

At nine, Jensen has turned philosophical. I imagine it's the age when kids start to question the world around them. With only one child, I don't have a basis for comparison. Jensen asks me about war, Hitler, how credit cards work. Why, if heat rises, is it colder on mountaintops? He asks the old questions, too: How does God decide on karma? Why did God make people? And I answer as best I can, but I often tell him that grownups have been asking these questions for centuries and that, for all the different conceptions we have of God, we can't truly know the mind of God.

After the loss of my third pregnancy, I remember asking: Why did I need to go through this? I'm not sure I have an answer, but one thing I didn't imagine is this: I could go through this experience without feeling terrible regret. Certainly, there are times when I feel melancholy. My son is growing tall and lanky. He is still happy and affectionate, and I have moments of feeling the way I did when he was small—that sense of preciousness, of time passing too quickly—but I don't imagine that having another child would mitigate this. Having two children would leave me less time to think about such things, but I'd still feel the ache of passing time.

When I reconsider my having thought "Life is chaotic, why not do it now?" I know that lots of people believe as I did, have children, and they weather those years, but my life isn't chaotic. I have time to notice the world as it's going by. I have time for the child we do have, and I suppose the best thing to report, contrary to popular wisdom, is that his childhood isn't going by in a flash. It's going by at just the right speed. I've had time to notice life as it unfolds, to keep trying to pay more attention.

A Globe of Light

Rochelle Jewel Shapiro

When I had my miscarriage, part of me thought I had willed the baby away. I was married and happy and by all accounts should have wanted this child, but, God forgive me, I didn't.

While I had never had a child before, I knew what it was like to be a mother and the thought of ever actually becoming one made my heart drop. I had virtually been a parent at the age of eight because I had had to raise my baby brother, Barry. Oh, my mother was alive and well, but as soon as I got home from school every day, she dashed out to help my father at his grocery store and wasn't home until nine. My two older sisters helped out for a while, but they were already in high school and had boyfriends and a busy social life and were soon going to be married.

Whenever Barry got the croup (which was pretty often), I was the one who had to turn the shower on hot and full blast and stay shut up with him in the steaming bathroom until he could breathe easily, never mind that I had carefully straightened my hair by rolling sections of it on Tropicana juice cans and now it would be a frizzy mop. Never mind that I got eczema from the heat and all that sweating. Never mind that my eyelids and lips got puffy. And never mind that after a few days, when his chest cleared, I came down with whatever he had and had to stay in the house some more.

One day, I sat on the carpet, looking at my brother through the bars of his playpen and I understood that we were both prisoners.

Even at sixteen, when most girls were dating, being a substitute mother was still part of my package. Saturday nights were big beer-selling nights at my parents' grocery store, so they stayed open until ten o'clock. If a boy asked me out, I had to drag Barry on the date, too.

To circumvent this, I began going out with guys who were nineteen or twenty, who could drive Barry to my parents' grocery store in Arvene, New York, a few miles from our house in Far Rockaway, where they could babysit him for a change. I fell in love with Bernie, the young man who was kindest about it. Not only did he gladly drive Barry to the store, but he played "read the license plates" with him all the way there.

"Why don't we take your little brother to the athletic field so we can pitch some balls?" Bernie suggested on our first date.

I was speechless with gratitude. The next day, he took Barry to the beach to dig for sand crabs and he also taught him to do a dog paddle in the water.

Whenever Bernie was expected, Barry would rush to the door to greet him and open it before I could. How could I not fall in love with a man who not only loved me, but loved my ball and chain?

Bernie and I talked about our future—the Tudor-style house we'd live in, the jobs we'd have. He loved that I was psychic, a gift I inherited from my Russian grandmother, my *bubbe* who was a healer. Bernie called me his "live wire," and encouraged me to use my talent as a career. "Someday, you'll have an office right in our Tudor house," he'd say. We fantasized about the places we'd travel to, but every time Bernie added, "And the kids we'll have!" I fell silent. I could foresee the ten-room house on a hill with a huge pine tree in the right-hand corner of the lawn. I could see the traveling we'd do, and I knew for sure that I was going to get married. I could see myself in a bridal gown, standing under the *chuppa*, the wedding canopy, but the only one whom I could envision at my side was Bernie.

When I was nineteen, Bernie took a small black box out of his pocket and handed it to me. When I opened it, there was a folded note on the black velvet lining. "One diamond ring to be picked out by Rochelle at Krasner's Jewelry," it said. I blinked at it. "Will you marry me?" he asked.

I got choked up. "Bernie, I'd love to marry you," I cried, "but I don't think it would be fair to you. I can tell you'll make a great father someday, but I can't wait to stop being a mother."

"It will be different with your own kid," Bernie assured me.

I thought of all the times my brother had wandered off at the beach, how my heart had pounded as I ran up and down the shore, calling out his name. I remembered all the days

I had to sit at home when outside, the whole of life beat like a pulse.

"Bernie, I'm so sorry, but I can't," I said.

He was quiet. I could hear his breath. He looked away from me, then back again. "Listen," he said. "There's no pressure. We'll get married and you'll see. Maybe you'll change your mind."

"What if I don't?" I asked.

"I'm marrying you for you," he said.

I sat there, gazing at him as if it were the last time I might ever see him. I loved his large brown eyes, his full lower lip, the set of his jaw, his dark wavy hair. I loved his broad shoulders and large hands, his humor, earnestness, and loyalty. No, I couldn't let him go. Maybe he'd be the one to change his mind and not want children. Or maybe I wouldn't be able to have them. After all, I had never been pregnant before. Everything would be all right, I told myself.

We were married that August.

To me, our marriage meant freedom. I learned karate. I took flute lessons and painted seascapes, all the things I couldn't do as a child. We did the traveling we had talked about. We went mountain climbing and river rafting. I could envision a whole lifetime of this and feel completely fulfilled. But whenever we saw a couple with small children, I'd notice Bernie looking wistfully at them.

Children were drawn to him. "How you doing, big guy?" he'd ask, ruffling a small boy's hair. And the next thing the boy knew, Bernie would magically pull a quarter out of the little fellow's ear. Then Bernie would look at me and smile hopefully.

Every night, when I put in my diaphragm, I was grateful that he never said, "Don't!" He never said, "Let's make a baby," even though I'm sure that he often felt that way. I would feel a twinge of guilt at depriving him of a son or a daughter, but still I didn't want a child.

Then, on our third anniversary, I missed a period. I wasn't always that regular so I didn't think much of it. But when I missed the next month, I got panicky. Every time I went to the bathroom, I hoped for blood. But there wasn't any.

"I think I'm pregnant," I told Bernie as grimly as if I were telling him that I had only seven more months to live.

Bernie lifted me off the ground and twirled me around and laughed. "I hope it's a girl with blue eyes and curly hair like you."

"Oh, Bernie," I cried. "I don't want it. I can't face being saddled with all that responsibility again."

He put me down and took both my hands in his. "You won't be," he promised. "I'll help you. And we can hire a great babysitter."

Babysitters! If I had bad memories of being a mother as a child, my memories of the babysitters my parents hired were not fond ones. There was the babysitter highly recommended by an agency, who stole my mother's jewelry, and the one who got a crush on my father and sent him a love letter. "That little hussy," my mother had called her. And there was a woman who got into my parents' liquor cabinet and fell into a drunken sleep, spread-eagled across their bed. At least she had been alone. Another time I surprised a babysitter in my parents' bed with her boyfriend.

"Babysitters never work out," I told Bernie.

But he smiled. "Of course they do," he insisted.

Abortion, I thought, the word flying into my head. But they were illegal then, and even if they hadn't been, could I have had the strength to go and do it? It was one thing to not want a child and another thing to get rid of it. I couldn't justify it to myself, especially not with a husband who yearned to have a child. I felt so stuck. I was in too much denial to go to the doctor. Bernie made the appointment for me.

Reluctantly, I went. I sat in the waiting room with women who were heavily pregnant, talking happily about what they would name their babies and what strollers to buy and where to get the best price on them and whether they would decorate the baby's room in pastel or primary colors. I thought of myself landlocked with these women in the playground someday and wanted to bolt. There were other women who had already delivered and had brought their infants with them in baby carriers. The amount of stuff they had had to drag along—two full shoulder bags of equipment—daunted me. I was the type who never remembered to bring an umbrella, and if I did, I always left it somewhere. It would probably be easier to stay home with the baby all the time, as I had with my little brother.

"Aw, you itsy-bitsy wittle coo," one mother said to her baby.

I could imagine my IQ dropping twenty points as well. I felt nauseous and I was sure it wasn't morning sickness.

When it was my turn to go in, I walked as if I were headed for the gallows. I told the doctor the date of my last menstrual period. I was hoping he'd say, "It's normal to be late.

Go home and don't worry about it," but instead he instructed the nurse to give me a urine and blood test.

For four days, I couldn't breathe, couldn't do anything but pray that I wasn't pregnant. I had almost convinced myself that I wasn't, but then the doctor phoned.

"You're definitely pregnant," he said. "About six weeks, maybe seven."

I felt as if the air had been knocked out of me. What would I do? How would I handle this? Why couldn't I go back in time and erase this?

He asked me to come to his office the following day. When the nurse showed me in, the doctor asked me to sit down. His brow was furrowed and the corners of his mouth were pulled down. "There's something else I have to tell you that isn't as happy," he said hesitantly.

I couldn't think of anything less happy than what he'd just told me.

"Have you had a rash or fever or swollen glands recently?" he asked.

"No," I said.

The doctor poked his pen at the lab result. "Your antibody levels show that you've had rubella sometime within the last six months."

"What's rubella?" I asked, terrified.

"You probably know it as German measles," he said. "It's a virus that's dangerous for pregnant women." He fidgeted with his pen. "It can cause birth defects such as blindness."

"But really, I haven't been sick," I said.

"Rubella usually lasts only three days and I've heard of

cases where the symptoms were so mild that the woman didn't realize she'd had it," the doctor explained.

My stomach clenched. "The baby will be blind?" I asked.

"It's possible," he said.

"But isn't there any way to tell for sure whether I had the virus during the pregnancy?"

Slowly, the doctor shook his head. "I'm really sorry, but there isn't." He was quiet for a moment. Then he cleared his throat. "Blindness isn't the only problem. There are worse things that can happen." He winced. "There can be liver damage and spleen and bone marrow problems. Sometimes there are malformations of the heart. It's not uncommon for the child to suffer stunted growth and mental retardation." He looked down for a moment. When he looked back up at me, a vein was ticking in his forehead. "I hate to say this, I really do, but it might be advisable to terminate the pregnancy." He clenched his jaw. "Shall I schedule a D and C?"

Stunned, I gripped the arms of the chair. This doctor was giving me permission—no, he was *advising* me to get rid of the baby. I wouldn't have to go to some back alley to get an abortion. But I couldn't say yes. I couldn't say no either. I was frozen.

"Well, think about it," the doctor said, "but don't wait too long."

When Bernie came home that night, I told him what had happened.

His face dropped. His eyes got teary. "Our poor baby," he said, and sat right down on the couch as if his legs could no longer bear his weight. "It's such a shock. Out of the blue like this when everything seemed so perfect." And then he reached out to me and sat me on the couch next to him. "I wish I'd been with you today. It must have been hell for you."

I sat there stiffly, ashamed at getting sympathy for a child I didn't want. "What do you want me to do?" I asked.

He rubbed the back of my neck. "Honey, I don't believe in abortions," he said, "except in extreme circumstances and this . . . this may be one of them."

"So are you saying that I should abort the baby?" I asked. I wanted him to take the responsibility from me. I wanted him to say, "Yes, this is what we have to do."

He leaned forward, elbows on his knees, and stared down at the carpet. "How can I make that decision for us? You'll have to come to terms with it. I'll go along with whatever you decide."

"But I can't decide, Bernie," I said. "If only I knew for sure that I had had rubella during the last six weeks, I'd definitely do it for the baby's sake. I wouldn't want to bring a child into the world that would have to suffer. But I don't know for sure when I had rubella and to me that means that I might be terminating the pregnancy for selfish reasons."

"Okay, you have a little more time to sort this out, but don't wait more than a week or it will all get harder."

I called my friend Toby for advice. "Don't you dare have that baby!" she insisted. "You never wanted a baby in the first place," she reminded me. "It would be extra hard to have one with birth defects."

My friend Jill said, "You must have the baby. You can't listen to the doctors. The same thing happened to my friend.

The doctors told her to get rid of the baby, that it would be deformed. That was seventeen years ago and her son just won the Westinghouse award for a project on conservation."

Night and day I wrestled with what to do. The week came and went. Another week passed. If I didn't act fast, I knew that my indecision would lead me down the road to motherhood.

But in my ninth week, I was in a ladies' room at Lord & Taylor when I pulled down my pants and saw it—a freckle of blood. The walls of the bathroom stall seemed to narrow. I began to sway and steadied myself on the toilet-paper holder. This was the blood I had been hoping for at the start of the pregnancy. Why was it happening now?

I went into the lounge and phoned my doctor, cupping my hand around the receiver so no one could hear me. "I'm bleeding," I cried. "What should I do?"

"That depends," he said. "If you don't want to keep the baby, just go about your routines. If you want it, stay in bed with your legs up."

Right then and there, I had a strong urge to start jumping up and down to try to end the pregnancy. But then I put my hand on my stomach and felt the faint swell. I thought about the baby inside me, the tiny fingers and toes, the eyelids just beginning to form, the buds starting where her teeth would be. I believed that the baby's heart was already beating and I suddenly wanted my baby to live. I went straight home, climbed into bed, and put four pillows under my legs. I began to fight for my baby's life as if I had always wanted it more than anything in the world. I got up out of bed only to go the bathroom. I drank beet juice to fortify my blood, as my Russian grandmother had advised women to do when they had bleeding. I wasn't hungry at all, but I forced myself to eat everything that was brought to me on a tray. I patted my stomach, just like the woman in the doctor's office, and crooned, "Aw, you itsy-bitsy wittle coo." I didn't care if my IQ went down *forty* points. Above all else, I wished that I'd one day sit on a bench in the playground with all those women, asking them what colors they had decided on for their baby's rooms, marveling over the strollers they had bought, and listening to whatever else they had to say, hanging on to each of their words.

After a week, the bleeding not only didn't stop, it got worse. I called my doctor. He told me to have my husband bring me straight to the hospital.

"The decision was made for you," the doctor said. "You already miscarried."

$\sim$

"You must be so relieved!" Toby said the next day.

As soon as she said that, I started sobbing and had weeping jags for days. I thought I had somehow harmed my baby by not having wanted it in the first place. I developed insomnia. Whenever I finally drifted off, I'd be awakened by the sound of a baby crying.

"It's a cat," my husband assured me. He brought me outside to show me the tabby and her kittens that he'd been feeding, but I couldn't be consoled. I stayed indoors. I didn't answer my business phone. How could I help my clients through their troubles when I myself was such a mess?

I didn't cook or clean. I was so depressed that I barely spoke to Bernie.

Once, when I saw him looking at my baby picture framed between my two bronzed baby shoes, I knew he was thinking of the baby we'd lost.

"Are you okay?" I asked him.

He straightened his back. "I'm fine," he said with a telltale catch in his voice. "And you'll be fine soon, too," he insisted. "It's just chemistry, all the hormones raging."

"If only there was a little grave I could visit," I cried.

"We don't need a grave," Bernie said, "We can say Kaddish for the baby together."

He put on a yarmulke and a prayer shawl. When I stood next to him, he put his arm and his prayer shawl around my shoulder.

"*Yis-ga-dal v'yis ka-dash, sh'may ra-bo,*" we chanted. Tears streamed down both of our cheeks.

That night, I still couldn't sleep. At two in the morning, Bernie found me wandering around the living room.

"Come to bed," he said.

I shook my head. "If I fall asleep I'll hear the baby cry," I told him.

"Don't worry," he said. "I'll be with you."

Finally, I lay down next to him, watching the clock for another hour until I fell asleep. A few minutes later, I did hear the baby cry. I opened my eyes and saw a tiny globe of light in the ether with the spirit of my *bubbe* and the five children she had lost during the pogrom. I began to sing the lullaby that Bubbie used to sing to me: "*Shlof, kinder, shlof.*" Sleep, child, sleep. And my own voice soothed me into sleep and my husband held me in his strong arms.

It was hard after that. I avoided the park where mothers were, and when friends and family asked, "Any good news yet?" I joked and said, "Yes, fruitcakes are going on sale." And yet, although the child had died, something new began to grow inside me, a yearning. I began to imagine what it might be like, a baby crying from colic, the constant flow of diapers, and instead of feeling horrified, I felt drawn. But was I longing for a new child or was I simply guilty about the old? I decided to wait. I didn't want to feel as though I were merely replacing the one I'd lost.

It took five more years for me to be absolutely sure. I had my daughter, and then, three years later, my son, and I cried when I saw them. Bernie had been right. It was different with my own children. There was not a moment where I ever felt as if they were my balls and chains. Each morning, I would be so excited to see them that I'd be standing at their cribs, waiting for their eyes to open. When they gave me their gummy smiles, I was overjoyed. I loved the sweet smell of the tops of their heads, the warmth of their bodies huddling against mine as I read to them, their sputtering and splashing in the bathtub. When they were old enough to go to school, I was the one who cried. When they left for college, I counted down the days until they would be back for holidays.

Sometimes, especially now that Bernie and I are empty-nesters, I think about the child I miscarried and wonder whether it had been a girl or boy and who it would have taken after.

Just the other day, when Bernie and I were driving to a

friend's daughter's baby shower, the newest kind where men are invited, he bopped his hand against the steering wheel.

"It just hit me that it's twenty-eight years since the miscarriage," he said. "We might have been grandparents today."

We were quiet for a few moments. Neither of us could look at the other.

And then Bernie reached for my hand and squeezed it. "We're so lucky to have our two kids," he said.

"Yes," I said. "And maybe those grandchildren will come, too."

"We won't forget, will we?" he asked, and I shook my head.

"Why would we want to?" I said quietly.

Then he turned and parked the car, and there we were, spilling out among all the parents, and parents-to-be, the grandparents and the kids, and for a moment, I felt that baby we had lost, that brief flutter of life, and then it was gone. I took Bernie's hand and held it, and we walked into the party.

The Road Home

Susan O'Doherty

August 1973

I am twenty-one years old, entering my senior year in college. I am conscious of my great good luck in having gotten this far. My parents aren't enthusiastic about higher education for females. They believe the money is wasted on a girl, who (God willing) will only marry and have babies anyway; in fact, they fear that an education will render me—already considered dangerously peculiar by my boisterous, athletic, beer-drinking, rampantly anti-intellectual family—stranger, less reachable, and ultimately unmarriageable. This is the worst fate they can imagine for me.

Because we are far from poor, I have been deemed ineligible for financial aid. Blackmailed by teachers, guidance counselors, and more liberal family friends, my parents have reluctantly agreed to foot most of the bill for the relatively inexpensive state college in Virginia where I am getting an astonishingly good education. They also pay for a dorm room and dining hall meals. For anything else (including the portion of tuition for which I have been granted a scholarship-related loan, clothes, textbooks, restaurant meals, alcohol, pot, bus trips to parties at other schools, and food and housing for those periods when the dorm is closed should I choose not to return home and work at my father's friend's factory), I am on my own. Since I feel I have been set loose in paradise—suddenly, my intelligence and interests, rather than isolating me, have marked me as a desirable friend and date; I am meeting fascinating, friendly people everywhere I turn, who share my passion for Joyce and George Eliot and who cheerfully confess to never having watched the Super Bowl—I am determined to make up for my dorky high school years by going everywhere I'm invited, trying everything I'm offered, and returning to the scene of my adolescent misery as infrequently as possible. Thus, I am in deep debt.

This summer, I am sharing a one-bedroom apartment with my two best friends, Nancy and SuSu. My job as a scooper at a strip-mall ice cream parlor barely covers my third of the rent, and we are not eating well. Friends come by to party on the weekends, bringing chips and dip, soda, and liquor, and these substitute for meals during the week. I gorge on ice cream during my breaks. My parents hope I will come to my senses, move back home, and attend secretarial school. Still, I am having the time of my life.

Until I discover that I'm pregnant.

The man I have been seeing (it is impossible to categorize him as my "boyfriend," much less "the father") is unsuitable in more ways than I can count: a thirty-year-old commitment-phobic keyboard player whose meager funds are allocated to the illegal substances he depends on to achieve the peak musical experiences that constitute his reason for living. We have been careful, but apparently not careful enough.

I don't bother informing him of my missed periods, morning queasiness, and thickening waistline. If he were to decide, uncharacteristically, to "do the right thing" and marry me, the scenario would be even worse than the more likely one, that he would say, "I'm with you, babe, but this is heavy. Let me call you tomorrow," and exit my life forever.

His very appeal, in fact, lies in his transience. All through my junior year, friends have returned from Christmas break, from spring break, from Valentine's Day and birthday dates, gesturing extravagantly with their left hands to ensure that the rest of us do not fail to notice and admire their newly twinkling ring fingers. They pore over china and silverware patterns, preparing to register at the "better" department stores. They talk about saving for a house with three bedrooms and a "rec room" for the kids, a backyard large enough for a swing set. These are the accoutrements of the good life for a woman in mid-1970s America, Betty Friedan and Gloria Steinem notwithstanding. I know that I am supposed to want them.

And I do want them, I tell myself. Just not yet. Not before I try out a few things for myself. Things like living alone, supporting myself without worrying about anyone else's needs. (Things like—this is in parentheses because I could not admit it even to myself—trying to be a writer.) Things you couldn't do if you had to put your husband through graduate school, as several of my friends are planning to do, or had to spend your days changing diapers and managing the laundry.

So I involve myself with impossible men: a married professor, a sadistic poet who continually rubs my nose in the perfections of his ex-girlfriend and my comparative inadequacies, and, most recently, my Jerry Garcia wannabe. If you asked me, I would tell you that I am in love with these men, with each of them in turn, and that the ambivalence is all theirs. And I believe this. When they behave characteristically, when they dump on me and then dump me, I cry. I listen to Crosby, Stills, Nash and Young's song "Our House" over and over, imagining the idyllic life we could have had, "watching the fire for hours and hours." It is safe to wish for this once they are gone. "He doesn't deserve you," my friends tell me in the wake of each desertion. Exactly. That was the point of him.

Except that now I'm pregnant, and alone.

My parents are not the sort to receive an errant (and now truly unmarriageable) daughter with open arms. They might allow me to move back home with a baby, but I would be reminded every day of their sorrow and disgrace. My life would consist of caring for the child (not, of course, a legitimate grandchild) and atoning for my sins, the chief of which would be considered to be my pride and arrogance in assuming I was destined for a better life than this. And I would never, ever get to finish school, would never get a chance to fulfill my secret, parenthetical dream.

Roe v. Wade was decided, definitively (we think), in January of this year. Abortion is now legal, if you can find a practitioner willing to perform one in this conservative state. And of course the operation is expensive. Still, it seems like my only option. My roommates and I make lists of friends we can hit up for loans, of fellow students who are rumored to have undergone the procedure and may be willing to share contact information. I am filled with dread, not for the baby, for I do not allow myself to think in those terms, but of the danger and the pain. Rumors still abound of young women with punctured uteruses left to bleed to death on filthy back-street operating tables by doctors who fear retribution. But if there is another choice, I don't see it. I begin another, secret list, of items (mainly my textbooks and some jewelry from my grandmother, my only belongings of any value) that I want Nancy and SuSu to have, "if anything happens."

So, when someone shoots off a cannon in my uterus as I bend over a barrel of mint chip ice cream, my heart fills with hope. The blood that first trickles, then gushes down my bare leg, accompanied by the blinding cramps, I take as proof that there is a God who listens to prayers. My coworker, a sweet-faced high school girl named Rhonda, ushers me to a chair in the break room and brings me a Coke. "Are you okay?" she keeps asking, as perplexed by my calm, I think, as by the condition I try to pass off as an extra-heavy period. "I'm fine," I tell her, and I believe this.

It's only afterward, as I lie on the couch with Nancy's heating pad, that I let myself ponder what it was that just escaped my body. I wonder whether it would have been a boy or a girl, what color its eyes would have been, whether it would have been an early reader, a queer duck, like me. I cry. I feel my heart is breaking. I really feel this. Like my grief for departed boyfriends, though, I can indulge in it only from the safety of the other side, when the danger of commitment is past. I think about this, too, and I wonder whether the baby sensed my feelings and sacrificed itself to them. I cry some more. I listen to Carole King belt out "Natural Woman," and I wonder what that is.

October 1986

I try to arrange myself on the minuscule chair in a way that communicates professionalism and seriousness of purpose. It's not working. Every time I move my legs they bump up against the knee-high table; to write notes I need to hunch over almost double. The graceful, fine-boned young woman seated across from me does not seem to have this difficulty. Her tasteful cashmere suit and perfectly coiffed hair contrast with my aging-hippie denim and single, sloppy braid. The briefcase at her feet is calfskin, as supple as her dancer's body.

I am her son's play therapist, and I have never felt so out of place in my life.

When this job was first offered to me, it sounded ideal. All right, not ideal. At this point, I've discarded the concept of "ideal." It sounded like a reasonable compromise: a position at a major university minus the challenges and rigors of an academic appointment. I could spend my days on an Ivy League campus, with an ID that afforded me access to the libraries, dining halls, and athletic complex, taking part in university life without actually having to test myself against scary demands and expectations. The only catch, as I saw it, was the population I would be working with: preschoolers with developmental delays. I imagined drooling, vacant-eyed little zombies and wondered how I could possibly relate to them, much less address their emotional and behavioral issues. But I figured it was worth a shot. Nothing else in my professional life was working out.

As it turns out, the kids are the one consolation here. They are adorable. Some of them do drool, and many aren't toilet-trained, but they are nothing like my mental picture of "retarded kids." They are original, funny, and endearing. They hug me just for showing up. The kids who are assigned to me—the ones with "behavior problems"—are the most fun. They are honest and brave. They hate the teachers. (So do I.) They find the daily routine repressive and stultifying. (Me, too.) They refuse to go along with this nonsense. (That's where I come in.) I understand them on a visceral, preverbal level. They trust me. We have a great time together, and I'm convinced that their play is growing richer and more creative each day. In terms of what I was hired to do, though—to teach them, through music, repetitive games, and structured role-play, to navigate their world, to express their needs and then meet them in responsible and socially appropriate ways—I don't have a clue. I'm trying to figure out how to do that for myself.

I am lost here. My entrée into the dining halls and libraries is meaningless, as I am not studying anything and there is nobody to eat lunch with. The students serve as a painful reminder of my own college days, when I believed I was going to make something of myself. I have nothing in common with them now. And as master's-level clinicians in an academic environment in which a PhD is the minimum requirement for consideration as a professional, the workers at our school are not looked on as legitimate faculty members.

I am lost within the school, too, among the teachers, therapists—occupational, physical, and speech—and administrators who constitute my colleagues. I had envisioned a circle of warm, loving, accepting souls, because, really, who else would choose to work with such children? And I had imagined myself being drawn into the circle, embraced.

It is a circle, all right, but a closed one. The kids are discussed as problems to be "remediated" through constant drilling, repetition, and haranguing. ("*Jonathan!* Can *you* put the *blue block* in the *red box?* The *blue* one, Jonathan. *Blue.* Look at me. *Blue.* Ba-*loo.* The ball is ba-*loo.* Melanie's shirt is ba-*loo.* Find the block that is ba-*loo.* Jonathan, look at me!" And when Jonathan loses it and heaves the blocks, he ends up in my office.) My first week on the job, a teacher referred a child to me because, she said, he was "exhibiting perseverating behavior." This was a three-year-old boy with Down syndrome who had never been separated from his mother before. He was picking up a toy phone and whispering "Mommy? Mommy?" into the receiver. I suggested that the child might be missing his mom. The teacher stared at me blankly and said, "Do you understand the concept of perseveration?"

I feel like a Martian, as if I were back in high school, where nobody spoke my language. When I talk about my previous job as chief writer for a highly publicized restoration campaign, my coworkers stare at me in disbelief, clearly thinking I am either lying or crazy. If I could do that, they in-sinuate, why would I choose to do this?

Because I'm finished with all that. I have given up on the idea that I will set the world on fire with my prose, and there is no other justification for continuing in the writing and ed-iting jobs that demand the twisting of my skills to sell ideas I don't buy myself.

For ten years, I held a series of increasingly lucrative writer/editor positions, eventually settling into a comfortable career writing fundraising material for nonprofit corpora-tions. I turned out to have a gift for this work, and I was highly sought after within the small world of educational and charitable development in New York City. The only problem was that I didn't believe half of what I wrote. Some days, not even one-tenth. These jobs had exposed me to the seamy un-derside of supposedly aboveboard organizations, and I turned out to be disturbingly competent at painting an attractive, impressive picture that glossed over fiscal misappropriations, cronyism, and incompetence. When a trustee of one organi-zation suggested that I had a future in the corporate world writing brochures and annual reports, I knew I had reached a major crossroad.

I had been justifying these jobs on the grounds that they supported my "real" writing, and that I was "honing my skills" for my great work. But the great work never material-ized. The "original" writing I did produce was shallow, deriv-ative, and glib. I wanted to blame my failures on my husband, Bill, or on the repressiveness of marriage itself, but in fact I had managed, while in my first job out of college, to find a loving, supportive man, who admired and encouraged my writing. It wasn't his fault that I was miserable, and making his life miserable, too. In the end, I had to admit that I simply had nothing of importance to say. And if that was the case, my day jobs constituted little more than shilling.

My friends have all moved on, have seemingly found their niches in life. Nancy and her husband, born-again Christians, are home-schooling their four children in the mountains of West Virginia. SuSu, a professional theatrical draper, and her opera-singer husband have embraced a sophisticated Manhattan lifestyle that I envy but can't emulate. I alone, it seems, was floundering. I returned to school for a master's degree, in the hope of making myself useful to someone else. Now, I am no longer looking for a calling, a vocation, just a reasonable compromise. There is no way to explain this to my colleagues, though. I'm as strange to them as I was to my family.

The mother sitting across from me is also having trouble figuring me out. All of the parents do. The high achievers, like this one, don't want to hear about how cute their kids are and how creative their play; they want to know what I'm doing to make them smarter. How I'm remediating the problem. The others, worn down by the needs of multiple children and the demands of the special-education system, seem to think I'm accusing or judging them when I talk about behavior issues. And each of them, every single parent, wants to know how many children I have. When I admit that I'm childless, any credibility I may have had is shot to hell.

Not anymore, though. I'm pregnant.

I've known for about a week. I haven't told anyone but Bill.

We've had too many disappointments in this area, and too publicly. After the first spontaneous abortion of my married life, my gynecologist, an elderly Teutonic psychoanalyst manqué, assured me that all was well with my plumbing and made frequent use of the term "hysteria" in suggesting that the problem lay in unresolved conflicts about my femininity. A few years later, another male specialist echoed his stance: "You career girls," he said, "bring these problems on yourselves."

Those issues are behind me now. I've given up any idea of a career, of personal achievement. The only thing that feels real to me, that seems worth investing in, is love: for my husband, for my tiny clients, and now, for my unborn child. I feel certain that I have resolved all my ambivalence and am ready to embrace motherhood and everything it entails.

And this job is ideal in one aspect: the schedule is perfect for a working mother. Many of my colleagues have children, and they talk about what a blessing it is to work school hours. My due date is in May, and the school is closed all summer. There is a daycare center right in the building, for when I return in the fall. And if, God forbid, the child is born with a handicap, I know now that it isn't the end of the world, and I'm aware of the available resources.

Although it is way too early, I stopped into a baby boutique yesterday and fingered the soft little onesies. I've started leafing through the parenting magazines in the school's reception area, surreptitiously because I'm not yet "out." And I have strolled by the daycare center and picked up a brochure, "for a friend."

I look at the mother sitting across from me, trying, I can see, to translate my enthusiastic gushing about her son's musical ability into something she can use. Next year at this time, I think, it will all be different. When she, or another parent like her, voices a concern about her child, I will smile knowingly and say, "I understand. I'm a mother myself." I imagine carrying the baby to work in a Snugli, visiting him during my lunch hour, or sneaking in to tickle her under the chin between sessions. I even dare to hope that motherhood will give me entrée into the closed circle of my colleagues, that the shared interests of *Sesame Street*, breast vs. bottle, pacifier vs. thumb, will draw me in as physical proximity and similarity of professional function have failed to do.

I shift positions in the tiny chair, and I feel a suspicious wetness as I cross my legs. I realize that the tugging sensation in my pelvic region is not merely the result of scrunching my body into impossible positions. I lose track of what the mother is asking me. I feel my eyes well up. I excuse myself and lock myself in the women's room. I kick the door. I stuff a hand into my mouth to keep from crying aloud, and I find myself biting down, hard. *You idiot*, I say to my reflection. *What the hell made you think you could pull this off?*

September 1991

The furniture I have brought with me from New York lends the apartment an unsettling, dreamlike quality, familiar and strange at the same time. The antique oak bookcases look misplaced, both in time period and in scale, in the low-ceilinged, aggressively modern living room. I'm sitting at my computer, staring out the window, just as I did at home, but the view—a lawn and trees rather than the gritty sidewalk and soot-stained brick I'm used to—induces vertigo.

Bill is here, helping me to settle in. He will fly back to New York tonight. Tomorrow I will begin my clinical internship in psychology at a veterans' hospital attached to a large university hospital in North Carolina.

I didn't have to move so far away. There are plenty of internships available in New York. Ostensibly, I chose this site for three reasons:

1. Bill and I have been planning to move away from New York for several years. An internship seems like the perfect opportunity to explore another area before committing to full-scale relocation.

2. My brother and his family live a few towns over.

3. I have become fascinated by the discipline of psychoneuroimmunology, the study of the relationships between mental and emotional states and physical health. This internship offers a rotation in PNI, with direct supervision by one of its leading practitioners.

All of these are perfectly plausible reasons for leaving my husband and home for a year to set up housekeeping alone in a strange city. But they're not *the* reason. I don't think I could even articulate *the* reason, except to say that I need a change: from New York, from my friends, from my daily routines, from my marriage.

I'm not looking for a divorce, or even a formal separation. At least, I don't think I am. It's just that, over the course of sixteen years of marriage, I have, despite all my fears and resolutions, become a Wife. We have slid, almost without noticing it, into the marital-roles trap. I feel middle-aged and confined. I want, just once, just for a while, to come home when I feel like it, and not be greeted with, "So, what's for dinner?" To eat a candy bar for supper if I want. To skip dinner. Maybe to skip coming home.

I will turn forty in March, and there is a major midlife crisis brewing.

Nancy's oldest, Katie, is applying to Bible colleges. SuSu's husband is in law school. There is movement everywhere, it seems, except on my doctoral dissertation. I am blocked. This strikes me as strange when I think about it (which I seldom do, because it makes my head ache and sometimes causes me to throw up), since I was known at my graduate school for being the one student who was never blocked. All the effort I'd thought I'd wasted learning to crank out prose on demand has been redeemed by the ease with which I'd breezed through papers, test reports, and psychological evaluations that had my classmates groaning and pulling all-nighters. I may not be the most brilliant theoretician ever to attend my school, but I am the champion word producer, hands down.

The topic I have chosen seems to me, and to my advisors, to be a perfect fit: the transformative effect of creative writing. I plan to explore the life and work of a novelist, Christopher Isherwood, using Erik Erikson's developmental stages, to show that writing can serve as a form of self-analysis; that it is possible to work out, imaginatively, on paper, issues with significant others from "real life," so that the effects carry over into our actual interactions with these others. I hope to demonstrate that the words we generate are capable of changing our world, of changing who we are in relation to the world.

I have done all the necessary reading. My thesis is clear and supportable. My dissertation committee is enthusiastic and helpful, as is my husband. And I can't write a word.

The fact that I have not written as much as a line of fiction or poetry for more than ten years does not strike me as a possible factor in my block. That is all in the past. I have found my calling. I remain an enthusiastic reader, and my clear, accessible prose style has garnered praise from professors and supervisors, but my creativity finds expression in other, more realistic, more adult venues now. I consider the therapy session to be a co-creation of therapist and client; we work together to reconstruct the narrative of the past, to alter the present in order to write a realistic, livable happy ending. I love my work. The idea that I am helping to write everyone's story but my own, and that this may not be the healthiest way to live, does not occur to me. When I try to think about the dissertation at all, I feel sick. I sweat. At the moment, I need a shower.

Bill's toiletry kit rests on the bathroom sink. It strikes me, suddenly, that he is a visitor here. That for the next year, when he comes, it will be as a guest in my home. I realize that he may be experiencing the same unvoiced frustrations and longings that have been plaguing me. His toiletry kit may well wind up on someone else's sink in the months to come. I've been assuming, without reflection, that whatever this is, it's *my* issue, something I need to get out of my system so we can get back on course. At this moment I see clearly, horribly, that by the time that happens, he may have moved on. This isn't a story I'm "co-creating"; this is happening to each of us separately, and I am not in charge of the ending.

As I step into the shower I feel a familiar cramping in my gut. I double over in pain and surprise. I had not imagined that I was pregnant again. A gleaming red blob the size of an eyeball drops down into the tub. I scoop it up and examine it. If I squint, I can almost make out a tiny shape, fishlike. I ease myself onto the toilet, shaking. I wonder what else has been going on that I don't know about.

July 1994

I lie prostrate on the operating table, my hands bound loosely at my sides. Behind a curtain hung so I can't see the lower half of my body, I can hear my obstetrician conferring with a nurse and various other green-swathed people who have not been introduced to me. There is an undercurrent of concern. I tune out their voices. There is only one voice I'm listening for, only one that matters.

And then I hear it: a repeated hoarse wail that sounds more like a quack. "Nothing wrong with his lungs," one technician says. I let out a breath.

He is real.

I moved back to New York more than a year ago. For the past eight months, as Bill and I planned, shopped, and decorated, rediscovering our early closeness through our shared anticipation and joy; as we informed family and friends of the impending happy event, I have been haunted by the idea that I'm making this all up, and that my intense wish that, this time, the positive early pregnancy test, the weight gain, the nausea, will result in an actual, live baby, has infected everything around me, including the ultrasound machines, with a type of shared psychosis. The fact that my due date came and went two weeks ago with no sign of labor did nothing to dispel my fears.

A month ago, I returned to my graduate school to squeeze into its cramped, airless conference room with the five long-suffering members of my committee and defend my doctoral dissertation. Amid the witticisms about my "productivity" and the triumph of delivering "two babies in a row," there were flattering comments from my committee members concerning the creativity of my thesis and the literary quality of my writing. My chair, a popular author in his own right, suggested that my dissertation was publishable, not just for an academic readership, but to the general-interest market, and offered me an introduction to his agent. (I knew this was nonsense, induced by the euphoria of finally being able to cross my name off the list of once-promising students who were at risk of never finishing, but it felt wonderful.) Guest readers inquired about my own creative writing. I explained, truthfully, that I had once written poems and short stories and even a play, but had ceased doing so for a long time, and that the process of writing my dissertation had put me in touch with a long unfilled need to write again. "A hell of a time to figure that out," my cochair commented, eyeing my bulging belly. I smiled and nodded, agreed that it might be a while before I was able to concentrate my thoughts in a sustained way, at the same time wondering whether this pregnancy was in fact my greatest fictional creation, a true triumph of mind over body. I lifted my glass of the celebratory champagne that traditionally marks a successful dissertation defense, but I didn't sip it, just in case.

The quacking continues, and I tune in to the comments of the green-clad crew. "Seven pounds," one says. I hear the hoped-for "twos" that signify passing marks on the Apgar scale of newborn health, and then the curtain parts and he is dangling over me. He stops crying and stares for a moment, then latches on to my nose and begins sucking. We all laugh. He is here. This is really happening.

Later, my obstetrician will tell me the reason for the hushed voices and the worry. "Your cervix and uterus are composed almost entirely of scar tissue," she will say. "Why didn't you tell me about your other operations?" There were no other operations. This is my first hospital stay since my own birth. The cause of the scarring will remain a mystery (my doctor suspects DES, but my mother says, "I have no idea. In those days, the doctor gave you medicine and you just took it"), but the mystery of the spontaneous abortions is solved. My son's birth will seem even more improbable, more miraculous, in this light.

Several hours later, I wake up from a deep, painkiller-induced sleep in a hospital bed, alone, with contractions so intense and painful it takes all my concentration not to scream. My stomach is flabby, but nearly flat. The baby, the Apgar scores, my husband's awed joy, must have been a dream. I have lost another one. There never was one. I ring for the nurse.

"What's happening?" I say.

"It's the Pitocin," she tells me. "You're on a drip." She explains that the IV I'm hooked up to is pumping the labor-inducing drug through my system to clear out any afterbirth. "It hurts, but it's nothing to be alarmed about," she says.

"The baby—" I begin, but I can't finish the question.

"The baby's fine. He's resting in the nursery until you're a little stronger. I'll bring him in first thing in the morning."

There *is* a baby. The baby is fine. I will see him in the morning. I roll up my pillow and clutch it to my chest, imagining that I am holding him. In between contractions, I allow myself to remember his round, bald head, his staring, intelligent eyes, and his perfect fingers and toes. I will hold him in a few hours. This is real.

April 2003

I am perched, once again, on a minuscule classroom chair. This time I am perfectly at home. I am the guest of honor in my son's fourth-grade class, invited to read my poems as part of a unit on composition.

At fifty-one, I am probably the oldest mother in the fourth grade. My husband and I don't volunteer to coach Ben's baseball and soccer teams. Strangers sometimes inquire whether we are his grandparents. When we visit Nancy, Ben plays with her oldest grandson. Well-meaning friends and relatives, ignorant of my history, have asked "What took you so long?" and "Don't you wish you'd gotten started sooner?"

For the first time since college, though, I feel I'm exactly where I should be. Parenting a creative, energetic, and demanding child uses up every bit of wisdom and patience I have accumulated. I could not have done this earlier in my life.

And, over the past few years, I've started writing again. At first I wrote for my own private pleasure; then, as my confidence grew, I shared poems and stories with my husband and selected friends. Last year I began submitting my work. I was not optimistic about its reception—the literary world had moved on without me, and the themes that occupy me now, primarily the passion and ambivalence of parenthood, lacked the grand sweep I had envisioned when I first set out to be an author. To my surprise, I have had some acceptances, including a few in journals I had dreamed of cracking the first time around. Ben, gratified by his immortalization in print, has alerted his teacher, resulting in this invitation.

When I'm done reading, the teacher opens the floor for questions. A serious-looking girl raises her hand. "You're a mother, and you're a writer," she says.

I wait for her question, but there doesn't seem to be one.

"That's right," I say.

She nods. "That's good."

I nod, too. "Yes," I say. "It is."

About the Contributors

Julianna Baggott is the author of the novels *Girl Talk*, *The Miss America Family*, *The Madam*, and *Which Brings Me to You* (cowritten with Steve Almond), as well as a book of poems, *This Country of Mothers*, and a series of novels for younger readers, *The Anybodies*, under the pen name N. E. Bode. She teaches creative writing at Florida State University.

Emily Bazelon is a senior editor at *Slate*, where she edits the magazine's health section and writes about law and ideas. Before joining *Slate*, she worked as an editor and writer at *Legal Affairs* magazine and as a law clerk on the U.S. Court of Appeals for the First Circuit. Her work has appeared in the *New York Times Magazine*, *Mother Jones*, the *Washington Post*, and the *Boston Globe*. She is a graduate of Yale University and Yale Law School.

Sylvia Brownrigg is the author of four works of fiction: a collection of stories, *Ten Women Who Shook the World*, and three novels, *The Metaphysical Touch*, *Pages for You*, and *The Delivery*

Room. Her works have been on the *New York Times* and *Los Angeles Times* lists of notable fiction, and she has won a Lambda Literary Award for fiction. She lives with her family in Berkeley, California, and in London.

Andrea J. Buchanan is the author of *Mother Shock: Loving Every (Other) Minute of It*. She is managing editor of *Literary Mama*, an online literary magazine "for the maternally inclined," and is also the editor of three anthologies: *It's a Boy: Beyond Snails and Puppy Dogs' Tails—Women Writers on Raising Sons, It's a Girl: Beyond Sugar and Spice—Women Writers on Raising Daughters*, and *Literary Mama: The Best Collected Writing from LiteraryMama.com*. She lives in Philadelphia.

Miranda Field's first book, *Swallow*, won a Katharine Bakeless Nason Literary Publication Prize in poetry. Her poems and reviews have appeared in numerous magazines and journals, including *Ploughshares, TriQuarterly, Fence, Boston Review*, and *Bomb*, and she has been awarded a "Discovery"/*The Nation* Award, and a Pushcart Prize. Born and raised in the UK, she currently teaches at the New School, and lives in New York City.

Pam Houston is the author of two collections of short stories, *Cowboys Are My Weakness* and *Waltzing the Cat*, as well as a collection of essays, *A Little More About Me*. Her work has appeared in many magazines and anthologies including *O* magazine, and her stories have been selected for the Best American Short Stories, the O. Henry Awards, the Pushcart

Prize, and the Best American Short Stories of the Century. Her first novel, *Sighthound*, was published in 2005. Houston lives part-time in the mountains of southwestern Colorado and is the Director of Creative Writing at the University of California–Davis.

Jessica Jernigan writes for a variety of publications. She's a frequent contributor to *Bitch* magazine, and she maintains a blog at www.jessicaleejernigan.typepad.com. She lives with her husband in Mt. Pleasant, Michigan.

Rebecca Johnson is a longtime contributing editor at *Vogue* and a mother of two.

Rachel Hall's work has appeared in a number of literary journals and anthologies including *Ascent*, *Gettysburg Review*, and *New Letters*, which awarded her their 2004 fiction prize. She has received other honors and awards from *Lilith*, *Nimrod*, *Glimmer Train*, the Bread Loaf Writers' Conference, and the Saltonstall Foundation for the Arts. She teaches creative writing and literature at the State University of New York–Geneseo, where she holds the Chancellor's Award for Excellence in Teaching.

Caroline Leavitt is the award-winning author of eight novels, most recently *Girls in Trouble*, a Book Sense selection. A book columnist for the *Boston Globe* and *Imagine* magazine, she is also the recipient of a New York Foundation of the Arts Fellowship, and was a National Magazine Award finalist and a Nickelodeon Screenwriting Fellowship finalist. She lives in Hoboken, New Jersey, with her husband, the writer Jeff Tamarkin, their young son, Max, and a cranky tortoise.

Dahlia Lithwick is a senior editor at *Slate*, where she writes about law and the Supreme Court. Before joining *Slate* in 1999, she worked for a family law firm in Reno, Nevada. Her work has appeared in the *New Republic*, *Elle*, the *Ottawa Citizen*, and the *Washington Post*. She is coauthor of *Me v. Everybody: Absurd Contracts for an Absurd World*, a legal humor book. She is a graduate of Yale University and Stanford Law School.

Jen Marshall is a writer and book publicist who lives in western Massachusetts. Her essay "Crossing to Safety" appeared in the *New York Times* bestselling anthology *The Bitch in the House*.

Joyce Maynard, a longtime journalist, frequent magazine contributor, and former *New York Times* columnist, is the author of the bestselling memoir *At Home in the World*, and six novels, including *To Die For*, *The Usual Rules*, and a young adult novel, *The Cloud Chamber*. For many years she published the nationally syndicated column "Domestic Affairs." The mother of three grown children, she makes her home in Northern California, where in addition to writing, she runs workshops on the personal essay. She can be reached through her website, www.joycemaynard.com.

Susan O'Doherty's writing has been featured in *Eureka*, *Northwest Review*, *Apalachee Review*, *Eclectica*, *Ballyhoo Stories*, *VerbSap*, *Carve*, *Word Riot*, *Style & Sense*, *Phoebe*, and the anthologies *It's a Boy* and *Familiar*. She is also a psychologist specializing in issues affecting writers, and has a forthcoming book on women and creativity.

Elizabeth Oness's collection of stories, *Articles of Faith*, won the 2000 Iowa Short Fiction Prize. Her first novel, *Departures*, was published in 2004. She is married to the poet C. Mikal Oness, and directs marketing and development for Sutton Hoo Press, a literary fine press.

David Scott's poems have been published in *Greensboro Review*, *New Delta Review*, *Madison Review*, and the anthology *Red, White, and Blues*. He has won awards in journalism as well as grants from the Delaware Division of the Arts.

Rochelle Jewel Shapiro's novel, *Miriam the Medium*, has been nominated for the Harold U. Ribalow Award in fiction. She's written about her adventures as a phone psychic in the *New York Times Magazine* and in *Newsweek*.

Susanna Sonnenberg's essays and reviews have appeared in *O*, *Elle*, *Parenting*, and *The Nation*, among other publications. A New Yorker by habit, she lives in Montana with her husband and two sons. *Her Last Death*, a memoir, is forthcoming.

Rachel Zucker is the author of three collections of poetry: *The Last Clear Narrative*, *Eating in the Underworld*, and the forthcoming collection, *The Bad Wife Handbook*. When not coparenting her two young sons, she teaches writing and is writing a novel. She also works as a birth and labor support doula. For more information, please visit: www.rachelzucker.net.

Copyright Notices